PHARMACOKINETICS AND PHARMACODYNAMICS

RESEARCH DESIGN AND ANALYSIS

Edited by

Randall B. Smith, Ph.D.
Director
Pharmacokinetics and Pharmacodynamics Research
Division of Medical Affairs
The Upjohn Company
Kalamazoo, Michigan 49001

Patricia D. Kroboth, Ph.D.
Director
Center for Pharmacodynamic Research
Assistant Professor
Departments of Pharmacy Practice and Medicine
Schools of Pharmacy and Medicine
239B Victoria Hall
University of Pittsburgh
Pittsburgh, Pennsylvania 15261

Randy P. Juhl, Ph.D.
Professor and Chairman
Department of Pharmacy Practice
School of Pharmacy
University of Pittsburgh
Pittsburgh, Pennsylvania 15261

A symposium held at the University of
Pittsburgh, May 16-17, 1985

HARVEY
WHITNEY
BOOKS

1986

HARVEY WHITNEY BOOKS
4906 Cooper Rd., P.O. Box 42696, Cincinnati, Ohio 45242

Library of Congress Catalog Card Number: 86-50775
International Standard Book Number: 0-9606488-4-4

CONTRIBUTING AUTHORS

Wayne A. Colburn, Ph.D.
Section Director
Pharmacokinetics and Drug Metabolism
Warner-Lambert/Parke Davis
Ann Arbor, Michigan 48109

Randall J. Erb, Ph.D.
President and Director of Scientific Affairs
Pharmadynamics Research, Incorporated
500 Sagamore Parkway West
West Lafayette, Indiana 47906

William E. Evans, Pharm.D.
Professor and Chairman
Department of Clinical Pharmacy
College of Pharmacy
University of Tennessee
Center for the Health Sciences
Memphis, Tennessee 38163

Thaddeus H. Grasela, Jr., Pharm.D.
Program Director of Pharmacoepidemiology
The Clinical Pharmacokinetics Laboratory
Millard Fillmore Hospitals
Three Gates Circle
Buffalo, New York 14209

Randy P. Juhl, Ph.D.
Professor and Chairman
Department of Pharmacy Practice
School of Pharmacy
University of Pittsburgh
Pittsburgh, Pennsylvania 15261

Patricia D. Kroboth, Ph.D.
Director
Center for Pharmacodynamic Research
Assistant Professor
Departments of Pharmacy Practice and Medicine
Schools of Pharmacy and Medicine
239B Victoria Hall
University of Pittsburgh
Pittsburgh, Pennsylvania 15261

Randall B. Smith, Ph.D.
Director
Pharmacokinetics and Pharmacodynamics Research
Division of Medical Affairs
The Upjohn Company
Kalamazoo, Michigan 49001

CONTENTS

FOREWORD

Problems of study design and statistical analysis are not new. However, the design, analysis, and interpretation of studies have recently become more complicated for pharmacokineticists. This is due to the renewed interest in assessing pharmacologic response in order to better define concentration-effect relationships. A symposium was held May 16-17, 1985 in Pittsburgh, Pennsylvania, to address design and analysis problems, particularly as they pertain to studies of the pharmacokinetics and pharmacodynamics of drugs. We hope that this book will be of value, not only to new investigators, but also to seasoned scientists.

The editors gratefully acknowledge The Upjohn Company for their support of this symposium, and the American College of Clinical Pharmacy and the Center for Pharmacodynamic Research, University of Pittsburgh for sponsorship.

The assistance of Brenda DeHaan and Joann J. Phillips of The Upjohn Company in preparing the manuscripts for publication is also gratefully acknowledged. In addition, we would like to thank Dennis Sinclair, Janet Kosko, and Susan Koett of the University of Pittsburgh for their assistance in effectively organizing the program.

Randall B. Smith
Patricia D. Kroboth
Randy P. Juhl

1. SYMPOSIUM INTRODUCTION

Randy P. Juhl

THE PURPOSE for gathering at this symposium is to examine issues surrounding the design and analysis of pharmacokinetic and pharmacodynamic studies. The participants of this symposium are here because of a common interest in the subject. In reviewing the list of registrants, there appear to be two major career paths that characterize the people in attendance. Some began as pharmacokineticists who subsequently developed clinical expertise, while others are clinical pharmacists first, who in later life studied from the gospel of pharmacokinetics. Given this situation, I thought it may be worthwhile to trace the parallel development of two disciplines, namely pharmacokinetics and clinical pharmacy, to see how they have come to have the common focus that we share today.

With your kind indulgence, I would like to draw upon some personal experience. In the early 1970s, I was a University of Iowa graduate student who continually demonstrated manic-like behavior patterns resulting from excitement over the emerging discipline called clinical pharmacy. During this time period I had occasion to spend an afternoon listening to Dean Emeritus Louis Zopf recall some stories from the good old days. Zopf related an incident from the 1930s when he was summoned to the newborn nursery at the University Hospitals to provide a consultation. A number of the infants were seriously ill with an unknown malady and as a last resort (some things never change), the pharmacist was called. Zopf's evaluation of the situation was quick and accurate. The difference between the sick babies and the well babies was diaper rash. An ointment containing a high concentration of phenol was being used on the infants suffering from diaper rash. He concluded that phenol was being absorbed through the skin and causing CNS toxicity, which resulted in the observed symptoms. The physicians thanked Zopf for his time and effort and then told him that he was crazy as a loon; drugs don't go through the skin! Zopf, knowing he was right, went back to his lab determined to show those hot-shots that drugs could indeed be absorbed through the skin. After some thought, he selected the rat as his test animal and strychnine as his drug. After shaving the backs of the rats, he applied varying concentrations of strychnine ointment to the exposed skin. Some rats died, others lived, and a portion of those that survived could be thrown into convulsions with a loud clap of the hands. The outcome was dependent upon the concentration of strychnine in the ointment. Eventually, the point was made and the problem in the nursery was solved.

The story was a fascinating one. As I started to thank Zopf for telling me this interesting story, he instructed me to be quiet because he wasn't done yet. He said, "The reason for telling you this story is so that you don't walk around thinking you invented clinical pharmacy. We didn't have a special name for it, we just called it pharmacy." He then went on to further elaborate on the difference between "invent" and "discover."

Zopf was right. The concept of the pharmacist dispensing information rather than solely a drug product is not new. In an essay on the development of clinical pharmacy, Gloria N. Francke described the early attempts to establish the concept.[1] In 1945 at the University of Washington, Professor L. Wait Rising developed a course wherein pharmacy students received academic credit for a controlled work experience in selected community pharmacies. Rising was attempting to develop an educational model in pharmacy that paralleled the clinical experience model employed in medical educaton. The visionary concept promoted by Rising was met with great opposition from one of his faculty colleagues, which resulted in resolutions by the American Association of Colleges of Pharmacy and the American Pharmaceutical Association condemning the new coursework. Heber W. Younken (a pharmacognosist) first used the term "clinical pharmacy" in 1953 to describe the Washington experiment.[1]

In 1960 a hospital administrator at Long Beach Memorial Hospital proposed a new type of pharmacy services. His vision was that by decentralizing the hospital's pharmacy services, more effective use of the pharmacist's expertise could be made. Such decentralized pharmacy services are now considered the optimal method of extending clinical pharmacy activity. Unfortunately, in 1960, the hospital's pharmacy staff opposed the concept and refused to be assigned to such areas.[1]

Given these two examples, it is a miracle that clinical pharmacy in the practice and educational settings was able to flourish as it did in the 1970s. Nevertheless, the discipline did grow. In the practice setting it was nourished by the emergence of drug information as a component of pharmacy services and the acceptance of unit dose distribution systems, which legitimize a more active role for the pharmacist in patient care. Long Beach Memorial Hospital became one of the shining examples of clinical pharmacy in the practice setting. In the academic arena, clinical pharmacy was aided and abetted by capitation funding from the federal government. As the discipline became more secure in its roles of providing clinical services and educating new practitioners, the need for a research component emerged. Even though research was an activity frequently disdained in the more formative years of clinical pharmacy, it is an integral component of the discipline today and one of the major reasons for the existence of the American College of Clinical Pharmacy, a cosponsor of this symposium. The focus of a great portion of clinical pharmacy research is pharmacokinetics and, more recently, pharmacodynamics. Thus, the interest of clinical pharmacists in the topic of this symposium.

As is the case with clinical pharmacy, we may tend to view the science of pharmacokinetics as a relatively new discipline. However, it is commonly thought to have had its formal beginnings in 1937 with the publication of two landmark papers by Professor Torsten Teorell. The term "pharmacokinetics" was first used by Professor F.H. Dost of Germany, who also published the first textbook on the subject in 1953.[2] Although many of the principles and the mathematical basis for pharmacokinetics were known for some time, the impact of the science in research applications did not occur until the late 1960s and early 1970s. The rate-limiting factor in the utilization of pharmacokinetics as a research tool was the lack of analytical methodologies with which to measure drug concentrations in biological fluids. As analytical techniques such as gas-liquid chromatography, liquid-liquid chromatography, and radioimmunoassay were developed for more and more drugs, pharmacokinetic investigation became more widespread. Today, analytical methods exist for quantitating nearly all drugs and the development of a pharmacokinetic profile is standard for new drugs. Thus, pharmacokinetics has attained a certain level of maturity over the past two decades in that it is widely accepted as a tool in promoting our understanding of drug action.

Unfortunately, pharmacokinetics is many times viewed as an end rather than a means to an end. Reports of increased half-lives, changes in volume of distribution, altered rates of absorption, and the like are not always accompanied by an answer to the question: "So what?" The clinician would like to know the potential application of a particular pharmacokinetic finding to the care of patients. The scientist desires a mechanistic explanation of the finding and its possible application to related areas of scientific inquiry. Some who travel on both sides of the fence see the need to answer "So what?" from both perspectives.

The search for the answer to "So what?" is not a particularly easy one nor is it a new one. Early in the growth period of pharmacokinetics, warnings were issued by prominent clinical pharmacologists who feared a proliferation of pharmacokinetic facts unaccompanied by data concerning their relationship to pharmacological effects. In 1975 Wagner acknowledged these concerns but stated, ". . . a major deterrent to such investigations is the lack of quantifiable responses in man. . . ."[2] Unlike pharmacokinetics, where advances in analytical techniques have fostered rapid growth in the discipline during the past 10 years, there has not been parallel growth in the measurement of pharmacological effects to spur the development of pharmacodynamics as a discipline. The rate-limiting step identified by Wagner 10 years ago remains a crucial issue today. Although we have made some progress beyond Zopf's model of strychnine-induced seizures in the rat, we still have much to learn in quantitating pharmacological response.

This symposium examines a number of issues surrounding the design of pharmacokinetic and pharmacodynamic studies. New techniques in design, data collection, and analysis are necessary in order to enhance our abilities to answer "So what?" For example, the practicalities of dealing with patient populations instead of normal subjects need to be considered in the design of studies (e.g., can a diabetic patient fast overnight and four hours after the dose as can a normal subject? Can I really expect to obtain urine samples every four hours from a group of patients who have end-stage renal disease?). The variables that must be controlled in a study designed to collect pharmacodynamic data are far more numerous than those in a straightforward pharmacokinetic study (e.g., do I need to include a placebo treatment to ascertain if reaction time fluctuates during the day unrelated to drug effect?).

Advances in computer technology and data analysis techniques present a good news/bad news situation. The good news is that data can be analyzed in an infinite number of ways with lightning quick speed. The bad news is that I don't have the foggiest understanding of triple randomized, complete block, crossover, ungrouped quadratic repeated measures industrial strength ANOVA with missing cells from page 391 of the SPSS manual. . . .but I got a p value of 0.001!

The speakers for this symposium have been selected because of their role in the continuing evolution of pharmacodynamic research. That is to say, they have made a sufficient number of mistakes to qualify as experts.

The purpose of this symposium is to share the experiences of a few of the thought leaders in the design and analysis of studies that examine the relationship between pharmacokinetics and pharmacological response from both the clinical and scientific perspectives.

References

1. FRANCKE GN. Evolvement of clinical pharmacy. In: Francke DE, Whitney HAK, eds. Perspectives in clinical pharmacy. Hamilton, IL: Drug Intelligence Publications, 1972:26-36.
2. WAGNER JG. Fundamentals of clinical pharmacokinetics. Hamilton, IL: Drug Intelligence Publications, 1975:1-3.

2. CONSIDERATIONS FOR EVALUATING DRUG CONCENTRATION-EFFECT RELATIONSHIPS

William E. Evans

CONSIDERATIONS FOR EVALUATING DRUG CONCENTRATION-EFFECT RELATIONSHIPS

William E. Evans

A DEFINED RELATIONSHIP between drug concentration in biological fluids and drug effect is a fundamental tenet for using pharmacokinetic principles to optimize drug therapy. Although monitoring serum concentrations has become standard practice for dosing many drugs, the extent to which drug concentration-effect relationships have been evaluated varies extensively among those commonly monitored drugs. Ongoing research continues to refine the mathematical approaches,[1] drug analysis techniques, and the physiological and pharmacological basis of pharmacokinetics and pharmacodynamics. However, drug concentration-effect relationships are usually complex and often population specific, requiring one to critically assess the context within which these principles can be rationally used to assess and optimize therapy with selected drugs. Several published studies have documented how this process can be beneficial, and selected examples of these studies are discussed in the following papers. Despite the strong theoretical basis and the intuitively sound rationale for applying pharmacokinetics to routine patient care, the process is not straightforward and may have considerable limitations under certain circumstances. Recognition of these limitations should lead to more appropriate clinical application of pharmacokinetics and pharmacodynamics, and should direct future areas of research. This overview will attempt to identify selected elements of clinical pharmacodynamics that should be considered when evaluating drug concentration-effect relationships. The overall goal is to develop a rational process for using drug concentrations, pharmacokinetic principles, and pharmacodynamic criteria to optimize drug therapy in individual patients.

Basis for Optimization of Drug Therapy

TOXICITY OR THERAPEUTIC EFFECT

With some drugs, optimization is accomplished primarily by minimizing the probability of toxicity; with other drugs, benefits are achieved by increasing the probability of the desired therapeutic effects. It follows, therefore, that drugs that do not produce toxicity at dosages or serum concentrations close to those required for therapeutic effects will not usually require serum concentration monitoring. For such drugs, it is common to use dosages high enough to ensure therapeutic concentrations in essentially all patients, since toxicity is of little concern. Conversely, drugs that frequently produce toxicity at dosages or concentrations close to those required for therapeutic effects are the drugs most commonly monitored and for which commercial assays are usually available. With such drugs, the target serum concentration range (i.e, therapeutic range) is usually small, necessitating relatively precise selection of the dosage schedule to be used.

THERAPEUTIC RANGE

The process of using drug concentration-effect relationships to optimize therapy is based, in part, on the premise that a concentration range associated with a greater likelihood of therapeutic response has been established. This drug concentration range is commonly referred to as the therapeutic range. However, the concept of a therapeutic range for serum concentrations of drugs is commonly misunderstood. Unfortunately, many inexperienced users of therapeutic drug concentration monitoring assume that the therapeutic range for most drugs has been well defined from carefully controlled clinical trials. Another common misconception by novice users is that once concentrations are achieved in the therapeutic range, the desired clinical response will occur. By developing a better appreciation of the drug concentration-effect relationships that define the therapeutic range of individual drugs, one can develop a more rational approach to applying pharmacokinetic and pharmacodynamic principles in clinical practice.

PROBABILITY OF RESPONSE

In general, a therapeutic range should never be considered in absolute terms, since it represents no more than a combination of probability curves. A therapeutic range is more appropriately defined as a range of drug concentrations within which the probability of the desired clinical response is relatively high and the probability of unacceptable toxicity is relatively low. This concept is depicted graphically in Figure 1 for a hypothetical drug.[2] As can be seen, the probability of the desired therapeutic effect is very low (i.e., less than five percent) when drug concentrations are low (i.e., <5 mg/L), as is the probability of toxicity.

However, it should be noticed that there is some small possibility of either the desired response or toxicity, even in the absence of a measurable drug concentration. This would be expected in a large study, assuming that some patients will recover spontaneously without any drug therapy, and some will develop signs or symptoms (i.e., adverse effects) that are unrelated but coincidental with drug administration. For this hypothetical drug, as concentrations increase between about 5 and 20 mg/L, the probability of response increases from about 20 percent to about 80 percent, then plateaus. Over the same concentration range, the probability of toxicity increases more slowly, from <5 percent to only about 10 percent, then begins to increase more rapidly as concentrations exceed 20 mg/L.

Thus, for a given patient, if one were given such data from a large, well controlled study of comparable patients, what therapeutic range would one use? If 10 mg/L was selected as the lower end of the range, then the minimum probability of response would be about 50 percent. If 20 mg/L was chosen as the upper end of the therapeutic range, then the maximum probability of response would be about 75 percent. Over this same concentration range, the probability of unacceptable toxicity would remain less than about 10 percent.

In this hypothetical example, the potential benefits of achieving a drug concentration in the therapeutic range are clear, since below this range the probability of response is considerably less and above the range there is a considerable increase in the probability of toxicity without any appreciable increase in response. However, it should be clear from this example that patients with concentrations below the therapeutic range may respond (5–50 percent chance), while those in the upper end of the range may fail to respond (25 percent chance). Likewise, toxicity may occur in those patients within the therapeutic range (< 10 percent chance), or may be absent in those exceeding the upper end of the range.

Unfortunately, concentration-effect charts such as those shown in Figure 1,[2] based on large numbers of prospectively studied patients, do not exist for many drugs. Moreover, with most drugs there are discrete subpopulations (because of disease, age, concurrent therapy, and so on) for whom concentration-effect relationships differ from the norm. Although it is common to find therapeutic ranges for many drugs, these target values are seldom described in terms of the probability of a specific common outcome being observed. However, based on clinical experiences with commonly monitored drugs, it is generally accepted that the probability of response is greater and/or toxicity lower if concentrations in the therapeutic range are achieved.

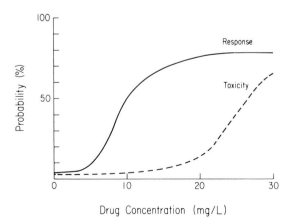

Figure 1. Relation between drug concentration and drug effects for a hypothetical drug (reproduced with permission from Reference 2).

Table 1. Selected Considerations When Designing or
Evaluating Clinical Pharmacodynamic Studies

Outcome Measurements	**Pharmacokinetics**
efficacy, toxicity	model
partial, complete	parameter (selection, estimates)
objective, subjective	metabolites
immediate, long-term	random effects (assay, sampling, etc.)
Covariates	**Statistics**
other therapy	model
disease(s)	time-effects
biological	covariates
environmental	sample size

Considerations for Establishing Therapeutic Range

To better define these therapeutic ranges, prospective, controlled clinical trials with objective outcome measures are needed. However, such studies often require a large number of patients, long follow-up periods, strict control of other therapeutic interventions, and appropriate study design and analysis to account for covariates that may also influence outcome (e.g., severity of disease, other illnesses, drug-drug and drug-disease interactions). Several of the important considerations are summarized in Table 1. Some of these considerations, such as drug-disease interactions, drug-drug interactions, pharmacodynamic modeling, and methods for estimating population pharmacokinetic parameters are reviewed in greater detail in accompanying articles.

EFFECT MEASUREMENTS

One issue worthy of brief mention is the appropriate time and method for measuring outcome (effect) in a clinical pharmacodynamic study. For some drugs, effects can be measured within minutes of drug administration (e.g., changes in FEV_1 following theophylline, changes in PR interval following verapamil). For other drugs, outcome should be measured after several days or weeks (e.g., antibiotics) or even years of therapy for some drugs (e.g., cure of cancer, chronic control of seizures). Moreover, for drugs such as theophylline that produce effects that are measurable immediately (FEV_1), one is often more interested in long-term measures of outcome when establishing a therapeutic range for chronic therapy (e.g., control of asthma over several months to years). Data that establish the probability of asthmatic symptoms and the probability of toxicity over a defined concentration range would be of greatest use to the clinician. The same can be said for several other drugs that are given to treat chronic illnesses, including digoxin, phenytoin, procainamide, and salicylates.

DISEASE, PATIENT, AND TREATMENT VARIABLES

Since many disease, patient, and treatment variables may influence the relationship between drug concentration and drug effect, the importance of drug concentration should ideally be assessed in the presence and absence of these other covariates. One approach to dealing with this problem is exemplified in studies of the relationship between methotrexate clearance (or Cp_{ss}) and disease relapse in children with acute lymphocytic leukemia (ALL) (Figure 2).[3] Our most recent analysis of these 108 patients indicates that the probability of relapse is significantly greater in patients who have steady-state serum concentrations $<16\mu$mol.[4] Since several other covariates are known to have potential prognostic significance in childhood ALL (e.g., white cell count at diagnosis, hemoglobin, DNA index, age, sex, and race), a stepwise multivariate analysis of Cox's proportional hazards regression model[5] was used to determine those variables with independent prognostic importance, and to determine whether methotrexate CP_{ss} retains its prognostic importance when the hazard of treatment failure is adjusted for the influence of other variables affecting outcome, including time at risk for failure.

This model can be used to estimate a ratio hazard function indicating the relative risk of treatment failure (relapse) in patients with concentrations below a predefined value compared to those with concentrations above this value. Likewise, multivariate analysis of Cox's regression can be used to assess the influence of drug concentration in a model containing other covariates that potentially influence drug effects. Although the proportional hazards regression model is suita-

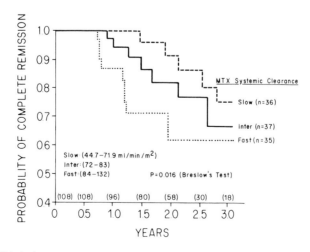

Figure 2. Relation between probability of complete remission and methotrexate clearance in children with acute lymkphocytic leukemia. Kaplan-Meier curves of complete remission in the three subgroups of patients according to their median rate of methotrexate systemic clearance. The numbers shown in parentheses represent the number of patients who have reached or exceeded the corresponding time from diagnosis (reproduced with permission from Reference 3).

ble for analyzing clinical pharmacodynamic data for drugs used in chronic therapy, published clinical pharmacodynamic studies using this approach are uncommon. One reason may be the logistical difficulties of such long-term studies and the uncertainty of when and how frequently drug concentrations should be measured to evaluate the relationship between drug concentrations and long-term effects.

TOXICITY AND TIME AT RISK

When assessing the relation between drug concentrations and toxicity, one often desires to estimate the probability of toxicity relative to time at risk, in addition to drug concentrations. Recently, Kennedy et al.[6] used a Kaplan-Meier analysis[7] to estimate the probability of renal dysfunction associated with cyclosporine therapy. As depicted in Figure 3, this analysis expresses the probability of renal impairment as a function of both drug concentration and duration of therapy, allowing one to estimate the relative risk of toxicity for patients in each of the three concentration ranges.[6]

Additionally, one could use the Cox regression model[5] to estimate the relative hazard of toxicity as a function of drug concentration after adjusting for other variables that may influence toxicity (e.g., other drugs, age, disease status).

Drug Concentration Monitoring

Once target serum concentrations have been established, the process of selecting the most appropriate dosage regimen to achieve concentrations in a relatively narrow range may be complicated by unpredictable intra- and interpatient variability in drug disposition.

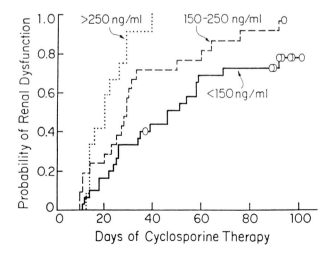

Figure 3. Relation between probability of renal dysfunction, serum concentration of cyclosporine, and length of therapy as reported by Kennedy et al. (reproduced with permission from Reference 6).

Appropriate application of pharmacokinetic principles, incorporating prior and subsequent measurements of drug concentration and effects, can improve the quality of dosage adjustments. Guidelines to this end have recently been addressed by Peck and Rodman.[1]

SYSTEMATIC APPROACH

Although a single "best" approach to using drug concentrations does not exist for every drug, it is imperative to realize that without a systematic approach to therapeutic drug concentration monitoring, drug concentrations may be uninterpretable, unhelpful, and potentially harmful. It thus becomes essential to recognize the key elements of applied pharmacokinetics and to develop strategies to perform and use them most effectively.

There are numerous drug, host, logistical, and analytical variables that influence the interpretation of drug concentration data: time, route, and dose of drug given, time samples (i.e., blood, urine, cerebrospinal fluid, and so on) are obtained, handling and storage conditions of samples, precision and accuracy of the analytical method, validity of pharmacokinetic models and assumptions, concurrent drug therapy, and the individual patient's disease and biological tolerance to drug therapy. As summarized in Figure 4, many different professionals are involved with the various elements of therapeutic drug concentration monitoring, yielding a truly multidisciplinary process.

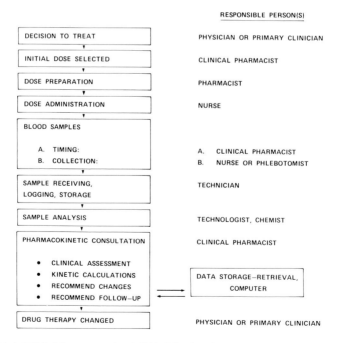

Figure 4. A multidisciplinary approach to individualizing drug therapy (reproduced with permission from *Aus J Hosp Pharm* 1983;*13*:107-13).

Since failure to properly carry out any one of these components can confound the assessment of clinical pharmacodynamic data and severely affect the usefulness of monitoring drug concentrations, an organized approach to the overall process is recommended. There is no single structure that ensures a well coordinated process for all drugs, since the organizational structure will have to accommodate the specific needs of each institution.

The organizational structure may even differ within a single institution, depending on the location of patients, special collection procedures for selected drugs, and the expertise and interest of medical, pharmacy, nursing, and clinical chemistry personnel. Regardless of the specific organizational structure selected, it should function in a manner that facilitates optimal performance of the individual components and it should routinely monitor the various procedures to document their quality.

Although some of the variables affecting drug concentration monitoring can be controlled or adjusted for (e.g., the accurate preparation and administration of drug doses), others are difficult or impossible to know or to control (e.g., individual differences in biological response to drugs).

These latter variables, which obviously have a major influence on individual responsiveness to drug therapy, are why drug concentrations are only intermediate therapeutic objectives and will not replace clinical response as the ultimate measure of success of drug therapy.

CLINICAL UTILITY

Given the rather large number of events that may have an impact on therapeutic drug concentration monitoring, one might question its value outside the strict controls of a research environment. Although the answer is probably different for each drug or drug class, intuitive logic suggests that drug concentration monitoring should be quite helpful for drugs with low toxic:therapeutic ratios and unpredictably variable pharmacokinetics. If one monitors and controls only the amount (i.e., dosage) of drug given to individual patients, variability in drug absorption, distribution, and elimination will influence the actual systemic exposure to the drug. By monitoring concentrations of drug that are attained in individual patients, one can modify therapy to adjust for variability in these pharmacokinetic processes. Thus, an appropriately obtained and measured concentration more directly reflects the amount of drug actually delivered than does simply the dose given.

It must be recognized, however, that drug concentrations in serum are generally not equivalent to drug concentrations at the site of action. It is simply assumed that they are in equilibrium with drug concentrations at the receptor and that there is a better correlation between serum concentration and drug effects than between dose prescribed and drug effects. These relationships have been defined more clearly for some drugs than others. For each drug, one should look closely at the definition of its therapeutic range, paying particular attention to the types of studies, patients, diseases, and measures of drug effects that provide the basis for each therapeutic range.

Summary

Pharmacodynamic data for commonly monitored drugs have been reviewed in detail and form the basis for a recently published textbook on applied pharmacokinetics.[2] When reading this material, one should look closely at how the studies were designed and ask the following questions: were they prospective, well controlled, and randomized? What type of patient population was studied? Did the patients have the same disease, concurrent therapy, age, and so on as the individual patient you are treating? Were the methods used to measure effects and end points the same as you are using? Was the therapeutic range based on an analytical method comparable in accuracy and precision to the one you are using? By answering these types of questions, one can more critically evaluate clinical drug concentration-effect relationships and more closely determine the extent to which a published therapeutic range can be applied in specific clinical situations.

This presentation and manuscript were adapted from a chapter entitled "General principles of applied pharmacokinetics." In: Applied pharmacokinetics: principles of therapeutic drug monitoring. Evans WE, Schentag JJ, and Jusko WJ, eds. San Francisco: Applied Therapeutics Inc., 1986.

References

1. PECK CC, RODMAN JH. Analysis of pharmacokinetic data for individualizing drug dosage regimens. In: Applied pharmacokinetics: principles of therapeutic drug monitoring. 2nd ed. San Francisco, CA: Applied Therapeutics Inc., 1986.

2. EVANS WE, SCHENTAG J, JUSKO WJ, eds. Applied pharmacokinetics: principles of therapeutic drug monitoring. 2nd ed. San Francisco, CA: Applied Therapeutics, Inc., 1986.

3. EVANS WE, CROM WR, STEWART CF, et al. Methotrexate systemic clearance influences probability of release in children with standard-risk acute lymphocytic leukemia. *Lancet* 1984;*1*:359-62.

4. EVANS WE, CROM WR, ABROMOWITCH M, et al. Clinical pharmacodynamics of high-dose methotrexate in acute lymphocytic leukemia: identification of a relation between concentration and effect. *N Engl J Med* 1986;*314*:471-7.

5. COX DR. Regression models and life-tables. *J R Stat Soc Br* 1972;*34*:187-202.

6. KENNEDY MS, YEE GC, MCGUIRE TR, CROWLEY JJ, DEEG HT. Correlation of serum cyclosporine concentration with renal dysfunction in marrow transplant recipients. *Transplant Proc* 1985;*14*(suppl 1):196-201.

7. KAPLAN EL, MEIER P. Nonparametric estimation from incomplete observations. *J Am Stat Assoc* 1958;*53*:457-81.

3. DESIGN AND ANALYSIS OF DRUG INTERACTION STUDIES

Patricia D. Kroboth

DESIGN AND ANALYSIS OF
DRUG INTERACTION STUDIES

Patricia D. Kroboth

DRUG INTERACTIONS have been a focus of attention for pharmacists, physicians, and researchers for years because of potential therapeutic benefits or problems that can result. Drug interactions can be due to changes in pharmacokinetics, changes in pharmacodynamics, or a combination of both. The ultimate importance of a drug interaction, however, lies not in whether the pharmacokinetics are altered by a second drug, but whether the response to the drug changes in the presence of the second drug. As researchers, then, the examination of a potential drug interaction cannot end with a pharmacokinetic study.

The discussion that follows is divided into two segments. In the first section, some well known examples of drug interactions and the designs of the studies that elucidated the clinical importance and the mechanisms of the interactions will be briefly reviewed. The second part of the discussion will address important elements of the study design and analysis.

Types of Drug Interactions

PHARMACOKINETIC INTERACTIONS

A typical relationship between drug effect and plasma concentration is illustrated in Figure 1. An equation for determining the magnitude of the effect resulting from a given plasma concentration of drug (the effector drug) is also provided in Figure 1.[1] Very simply, once this relationship has been defined, the theoretical magnitude of effect can be determined for any plasma concentration. When plasma concentrations are altered, the magnitude of the effect will be altered. This occurs when the dose is changed or when therapy with an interactor drug is started. For example, if an interactor drug decreases clearance and thus increases plasma concentrations of the effector drug, there will be a concomitant increase in effect. The magnitude of the observed change in effect depends on which part of the curve concentrations fall before therapy with the interactor drug. The greatest change in observed effect occurs when concentrations of the effector drug are in the range that causes 20 to 80 percent of maximum effect.

However, factors other than plasma concentrations of the effector drug also influence the clinical importance of kinetic interactions. The most obvious of these is the safety margin of the effector drug. In addition, plasma concentrations of the interactor drug, stereoisomers of the effector drug, and active metabolites can also be important for some drug-drug interactions.

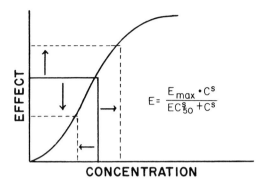

Figure 1. Effect-concentration curve demonstrating a relationship between an observed effect and plasma concentration. This example depicts how pharmacokinetic interactions can result in altered effect.

Concentration Dependence. When evaluating the clinical importance of a kinetic interaction, plasma concentrations of both the effector and the interactor drugs can be important. This becomes even more apparent when plasma concentrations of the interactor following oral administration are variable, e.g., the interaction between theophylline (the effector) and erythromycin (the interactor).

In 1977, Kozak et al. first reported that five asthmatic patients on chronic theophylline therapy developed nausea and vomiting approximately 36–48 hours after starting therapy with erythromycin. Plasma theophylline concentrations obtained during erythromycin therapy were higher than those prior to concomitant therapy.[2] Subsequently, several studies of this drug interaction appeared in the literature.[3-5] Some found statistical significance of this drug interaction, others did not. However, decreases in plasma theophylline clearance as large as 50 percent were noted.[3] The reason for this variability in results was elusive, but was finally explained by Prince and coworkers who evaluated plasma concentrations of both erythromycin and theophylline. They demonstrated a linear relationship between peak erythromycin concentration and percent change in theophylline clearance. The higher the peak erythromycin concentration, the greater the decrease in theophylline clearance.[6]

Thus, this kinetic interaction demonstrates that evaluation of plasma concentrations of both the effector and the interactor can provide insight to the variability of a drug interaction. Furthermore, with respect to clinical importance of an interaction to individual patients, examination of the range of clearance values observed in a given study may be more meaningful than statistical significance of the change in clearance.

However, in order to determine whether a change in clearance of the effector drug is dependent on concentrations of the interactor drug, assays for both drugs must be available. This is not always the case. An alternative way of evaluating concentration dependency of kinetic interactions is to give the interactor drug in several different doses and then evaluate the kinetics of the effector drug.

This type of evaluation was done in a study of atenolol (the effector) kinetics following different doses of ampicillin (the interactor). The investigators administered atenolol 50 mg po alone, with ampicillin 1 g, or with ampicillin 250 mg followed by further dosages at 3, 9, 13, and 24 h postatenolol. The result was three different plasma atenolol concentration-time curves, which demonstrates the effect of dose (and presumably concentration) of the interactor on the effector drug area under the plasma concentration curve and clearance.[7]

Role of Stereoisomers. The importance of stereoisomers can be appreciated from a historical review of the drug interaction between phenylbutazone and warfarin. One of the first reports of this drug interaction appeared in 1967 when investigators reported that the half-life of warfarin was shorter when phenylbutazone was coadministered. However, the authors were puzzled by an increase in prothrombin time despite lower plasma warfarin concentrations. Although phenylbutazone displaced warfarin from albumin binding sites, increased free fraction did not explain the enhanced warfarin activity since the effect on prothrombin time persisted as long as phenylbutazone was administered. Thus, phenylbutazone altered warfarin kinetics, but the mechanism of enhanced warfarin activity was elusive.[8]

Warfarin, however, is administered as a racemic mixture. In 1974, a study of the two isomers in man demonstrated that not only is the S– isomer the more potent of the two, it also has the shorter half-life.[9] Later, when a stereospecific assay was developed, the drug interaction was reevaluated and explained. The phenylbutazone effect on plasma warfarin clearance is stereospecific.[10] Half-life and plasma concentrations of the S– enantiomer, the more active of the two, increase during phenylbutazone treatment, while total plasma concentrations of the R + isomer decrease. Although peak unbound concentrations of both warfarin isomers increase, the resulting unbound S– area under the curve (AUC) increases four-fold due to change in clearance.

The initial report of this interaction suggested that kinetics were not responsible for the enhanced prothrombin response. However, examination of the phenylbutazone effect on the individual stereoisomers demonstrated that the increase in prothrombin time was due to an increase in free plasma concentrations of the active isomer.

PHARMACODYNAMIC INTERACTIONS

A second type of interaction is the dynamic interaction. Addition of an interactor drug may cause little or no change in plasma concentrations of the effector drug, but may cause a change in the effect-concentration relationship. Figure 2 shows the most simplistic form of this drug interaction. If the interaction results in a curve shift to the right, the effect resulting from a given plasma concentration decreases. The opposite is true for a shift to the left. Dynamic interactions can also result in changes in slope (EC_{50}), or in the maximum observable response (E_{max}). These alterations may be due to interactions at the receptor site, changes in the receptor itself, or alteration in an effect that is mediated through two different mechanisms.

Dynamic interaction studies have two obvious requirements. First, the dose of the effector drug must be large enough to elicit a quantifiable response. This is described in the section on pharmacokinetic/pharmacodynamic interactions. Secondly, the effector drug must produce a response that can be reliably measured.

Reliable Response Measurement. The drug interaction between warfarin and disulfiram is an example of this requirement. Warfarin, the effector drug, produces a response (increase in prothrombin time) that can be reliably measured. When disulfiram (interactor drug) is added, the hypoprothrombinemic effect of warfarin is enhanced.[11] Since disulfiram does not produce changes in warfarin kinetics that explain the increased response, the drug interaction appears to be mediated through some effect of disulfiram on prothrombin or on hepatocytes responsible for production of coagulation factors. This drug interaction also underscores the importance of including dynamic as well as kinetic assessments when evaluating a potential interaction between two drugs.

PHARMACOKINETIC/PHARMACODYNAMIC INTERACTIONS

The third category of drug interactions, pharmacokinetic/pharmacodynamic, is the most complex. From Figures 3–6, we can see some of the possibilities. The first is a kinetic interaction, which results in increased plasma concentrations of the effector drug; and a dynamic interaction, which enhances response to the effector drug. The result is a large increase in response to the effector drug. The second possibility is a decrease in plasma concentrations and dynamics, resulting in a large decrease in response to the effector drug. Other possibilities are kinetic interactions that increase (decrease) effector drug concentration and dynamic interactions that decrease (increase) effector drug response. These latter possibilities may result in little change in response.

The following are two examples of kinetic/dynamic interactions. The first and perhaps the most often reported interaction in the last six years is the one between digoxin and quinidine. Several early studies

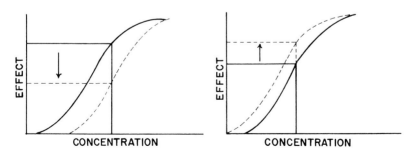

Figures 2a and 2b. Effect-concentration curves that simplistically demonstrate pharmacodynamic interactions. Drug interactions can result in a change in effect without demonstrable changes in plasma concentrations.

in man were purely kinetic, and demonstrated that quinidine (the inter-actor) decreased digoxin (the effector) clearance and resulted in increased plasma digoxin concentrations. Subsequent work in animals demonstrated that quinidine displaced digoxin from tissue binding sites. This suggests that despite the increase in plasma digoxin concentrations, less digoxin is bound to tissue sites where it is active. Because of the possible disturbance of the concentration/effect relationship, the inter-action no longer appears to be a simple kinetic one. It seems that there may be large increases in plasma concentration, but relatively smaller increases in effect, as simplistically depicted in Figure 5. Although the true clinical implication is yet to be determined, a recent study of the kinetics and dynamics of the interaction in normal volunteers did not support the current practice of decreasing the digoxin dose when quini-dine is added to the therapeutic regimen.[12]

A second interaction also demonstrates that a kinetic alteration may not lead to the expected change in effect. Oral contraceptives (OCs) have been reported to impair oxidative metabolism and to enhance glucuronidation of drugs. Because some benzodiazepines are metabo-lized through oxidation, and others through glucuronidation, they are an interesting family of drugs to use in evaluating the effect of OCs on drug metabolism.

We evaluated the kinetics[13] and dynamics[14] of four benzodiazepines: alprazolam and triazolam, which are metabolized oxidatively; and lorazepam and temazepam, which are metabolized by glucuronidation. Table 1 summarizes our findings. For alprazolam and triazolam, there were decreases in clearance and increases in C_{max} values in the OC sub-jects. The maximum psychomotor performance impairment was also greater in the OC subjects. At first glance, it may appear that the change in kinetics is reflected in the change in psychomotor performance. How-ever, even though OCs produced an increase in lorazepam clearance, the OC subjects experienced greater performance impairment than con-trol women. Furthermore, when E_{max} was corrected for differences in C_{max}, women taking OCs experienced greater psychomotor impairment following single oral doses of benzodiazepines. Thus, women taking

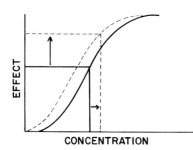

Figure 3. A kinetic interaction that results in decreased plasma concentrations and a dynamic interaction that decreases the EC_{50}; the result is a large increase in observed effect.

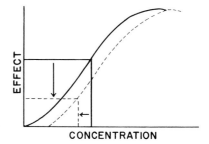

Figure 4. A kinetic interaction that results in decreased plasma concentrations and a dynamic interaction that increases the EC_{50}; the result is a large decrease in observed effect.

Table 1. Benzodiazepine-Oral Contraceptive Interaction*

	CLEARANCE	PEAK PLASMA CONCENTRATION	MAXIMUM EFFECT (E_{max})†	CORRECTED E_{max}
Alprazolam	0.8	1.2	1.7	1.7
Triazolam	0.8	1.1	1.3	1.4
Lorazepam	1.2	1.1	1.5	1.7
Temazepam	1.8	0.8	NE	NE

*Ratio of means (oral contraceptive/control).
†Decrease in psychomotor performance.
NE = effect not able to be evaluated. See text.

OCs seem to have altered benzodiazepine pharmacokinetics, the direction of alteration being dependent on route of metabolism. However, regardless of the direction of kinetic change, women taking OCs appear to be more sensitive to the pharmacologic effects of single oral doses of benzodiazepines.

Size of Effector Drug Dose. It should be noted that psychomotor performance data from the temazepam treatment are not presented in Table 1. The first requirement for dynamic studies, that the size of the effector drug dose be large enough to elicit an observable response, was not met for temazepam. Following administration of a single dose of temazepam 30 mg, >60 percent of the subjects experienced <15 percent decrease in psychomotor performance. Therefore, because the recommended hypnotic dose did not elicit a measurable response in the majority of subjects, the data were not evaluable.

The warfarin-disulfiram study described previously provides an example of the size of dose needed for dynamic studies. The warfarin dose administered is notably large (1.5 mg/kg). For a person weighing 70 kg, this 1.5 mg/kg dose represents warfarin 105 mg as a single oral dose.[11] This warfarin dose was used not only in this drug interaction study, but in many other dynamic studies done by the same group of investigators.

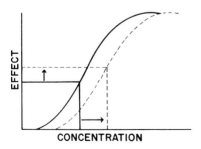

Figure 5. A combination of kinetic and dynamic effects in which a relatively large increase in concentration produces a relatively small increase in effect.

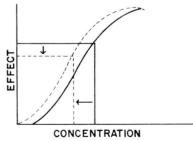

Figure 6. A kinetic/dynamic interaction in which a relatively large decrease in concentration results in a small decrease in effect.

Warfarin dynamic interaction studies are not the only ones in which relatively large doses are administered. Another example is provided by Ellinwood and coworkers who evaluated psychomotor impairment following three different doses of diazepam. The highest dose administered was 0.28 mg/kg po. This dose is diazepam 19.6 mg/70 kg body weight.[15]

Thus, there are two important lessons to be learned from these kinetic/dynamic interaction studies. First, a change in kinetics does not necessarily result in the expected change in effect. Secondly, when evaluating pharmacologic response, you must give a dose large enough to obtain an evaluable pharmacologic response. Failure to give a large enough dose can lead to incorrect conclusions or failure to answer the question.

EVALUATION OF DRUG INTERACTIONS

The following are some practical factors to consider when designing drug interaction studies:

1. Kinetic evaluation alone does not provide information about the clinical importance of an interaction. Because the interactor drug can influence not only the kinetics of the effector drug, but also the effect-plasma concentration relationship, measures of response should be evaluated.

2. Based on the few drug interactions reviewed, it is apparent that thorough evaluation of the clinical significance and mechanism of an interaction may take several studies. Planning a sequence of studies to appropriately evaluate the potential interaction is preferable to trying to answer all questions (and potentially answer none) in one cumbersome study. In addition, evaluation in patients may be necessary, as discussed by Smith.[16]

3. Conducting a pilot study to determine the dose required to obtain observable effects is time well invested. Although the importance of dose size was demonstrated in the kinetic interaction between erythromycin and theophylline, it becomes even greater for pharmacodynamic studies. Failure to give a large enough dose can lead to incorrect conclusions or failure to meet the objectives of the study.

Although some practical aspects have been addressed, the question of how to best design and analyze data from a drug interaction study is still unanswered. Like many questions, it does not have an easy answer. When reviewing the literature, you will find that much has been written about experimental design and statistical analysis, but little of this has been directed toward evaluation of drug interactions.

Elements of Study Design and Analysis

DESIGNING DRUG INTERACTION STUDIES

To determine the current standard of practice for conducting drug interaction studies, I surveyed the 1984 volumes of two prominent clinical pharmacology journals. Table 2 illustrates that a substantial portion of the current literature is dedicated to the evaluation of drug

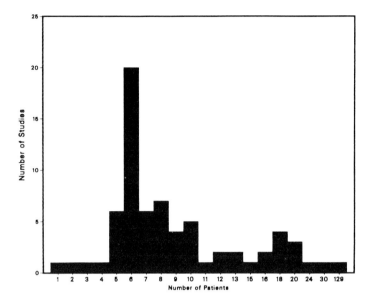

Figure 7. Number of patients evaluated in 70 drug interaction studies reported in 1984 in two clinical pharmacology journals. Note that the number of patients per study, presented on the x-axis, is not a continuous linear scale.

interactions. Of the 477 original articles appearing in the two selected journals, 14.9 percent were reports of drug interaction studies.

Of the 71 drug interaction studies, astoundingly few included evaluation of both the kinetic and dynamic aspects of the interaction. When only one aspect was evaluated, in the majority of cases (76.4 percent), it was the kinetic interaction that was assessed. Although a kinetic study may be a reasonable first step, potential problems with that approach should be obvious from some of the examples provided in the previous section.

Number of Subjects and Calculation of Power. Evaluation of kinetic studies in the elderly has demonstrated that results may be nonrepresentative of the general population when the sample size is small.[16] However, sample size is also important because it is one of the factors that determines the power of a statistical test to detect a difference if there is one. Figure 7 summarizes the number of patients included in 70 of the 71 drug interaction studies. Twenty of the seventy-one studies used only six subjects, with 74.3 percent including ten or fewer subjects. Although it is hard to believe, the authors of one drug interaction study failed to report the number of subjects assessed.

Table 2 also includes a summary of the number of trials with a "negative" outcome, i.e., trials that failed to detect a difference. Approximately 40 percent of the kinetic interaction studies showed that the kinetics of the effector drug were unchanged by the interactor. However, unless the investigators determined that the trial had sufficient statistical power (e.g., at least 80 percent power to detect a 20 percent difference), a negative outcome only means that the data failed to show a difference; it does not necessarily mean that kinetics are unchanged by the interactor drug. Of all the articles that reported a negative outcome, only one included data on the power of the study.

Lack of power may be even more critical for dynamic studies. Of 37 drug-drug interactions that included effect evaluations, there was no difference detected in 23 (62.2 percent). In 7 of these 23 (30.4 percent), there was a trend toward a statistical difference. However, the authors stated that with more subjects, the power would have increased and perhaps a statistical difference would have been found.

The problem of lack of power is not unique to drug interaction studies. In 1978, Freiman et al. determined that in 71 efficacy studies that had a negative outcome, a major problem was that too few patients were evaluated. Only seven percent of the studies with a negative outcome had an 80 percent probability of detecting a 25 percent difference if there was one.[17]

Table 2. Summary of Drug Interaction Studies Published in Two Journals During 1984

	NUMBER
Total Number of Original Articles Published	477
Drug interaction articles	71
interactions evaluated: 125	
antipyrine interactions: 8	
Articles describing:	
kinetic studies	42
dynamic studies	13
kinetic and dynamic studies	15
kinetic in normals, dynamics in patients	1
Statistical outcome	
kinetic interactions evaluated	96
no statistical significance: 38	
dynamic evaluation	37
no statistical significance: 23	
trend present: 7	
negative trials, power reported: 1	
Classification of designs described in the 71 articles	
crossover	64
parallel	7
randomized	29
partially randomized	1
randomization unclear	4
no randomization	37
blinded	9
no blinding	62
multiple-dose/single-dose design	37
single dose	14
multiple dose	20
Subject population evaluated in the article	
patients	15
normal volunteers	56

But, specifically, how does the number of patients influence power? Most statistics texts discuss power and describe it $(1-\beta)$, but relatively few provide a working formula and corresponding table or graph. The easiest way is to calculate ϕ^2. The formula provided by Dixon and Massey is:

$$POWER$$
$$\phi^2 = \Sigma_{i=1}^k \frac{(\overline{x}_i - \overline{\overline{x}})^2/k}{s^2/n}$$

where $\overline{x}_i$ = mean for treatment i, $\overline{\overline{x}}$ = mean for all treatments, k = number of treatments, s^2 = residual mean square error, and n = number of subjects.[18] All factors from the right of the equal sign are readily available from the analysis of variance (ANOVA) table. Power is determined by taking the square root of ϕ^2, and using the appropriate table[19] or power curves.[18] The larger the ϕ, the higher the power. From this equation, it is readily apparent that by increasing the number of subjects, both the ϕ^2 and power increase. Power to detect a difference can also be increased by decreasing the residual error, i.e., the amount of unexplained variability in data.

Blinding, Placebo Treatments, and Randomization. In evaluating efficacy studies performed in Europe, Bland et al. reported that a majority of the studies were double blind, randomized, and controlled.[20] Data from the current standard of practice survey (Table 2) make it obvious that this is not the case for drug interaction studies. This is unfortunate, because use of these techniques can help prevent the introduction of systematic bias. The importance of blinding and use of placebo comparison groups in studies that include response assessments cannot be overemphasized.

Randomization is also important for kinetic as well as dynamic studies. An example of our own work demonstrates this point. Several years ago, we conducted a study in which the primary objective was to define the kinetics of triazolam in dialysis patients. A second objective was to examine the effect of aluminum hydroxide gel on triazolam absorption. Because of practical considerations, it was decided not to randomize the trial. All patients received triazolam week 1, and triazolam plus aluminum hydroxide gel on week 2. AUC and C_{max} values observed when aluminum hydroxide gel was administered with triazolam were approximately 1.5 times as large as in the triazolam alone treatment. There is a logical explanation for these findings.[21] However, we cannot rule out the possibility that some factor other than aluminum hydroxide administration changed systematically from week 1 to week 2, which could also account for the observations. Had we varied the order of treatment randomly and obtained the same results, we would know conclusively that aluminum hydroxide gel was responsible for the increased AUC.

Parallel vs. Crossover Design. Spilker describes some variations in the design of both parallel and crossover studies. Although most drug interaction studies in the 1984 survey were done using crossover design, each type has its advantages.[22]

Parallel Design. In parallel studies, subjects are randomized to one of the treatment groups. Since subjects do not participate in all treatments, this may be the more practical design for certain types of drug interaction studies. For example, evaluation of the effect of OCs on lorazepam kinetics and dynamics would be relatively easily accomplished in a parallel design study by administering lorazepam to women taking OCs and a comparable control group. A crossover study would be difficult because of the problem of recruiting women who would participate once while taking OCs, and once while contraceptive-free for several months.

Data Analysis for Parallel Design. If the assumptions underlying parametric tests are met, data should be evaluated by either a Student's *t*-test for unpaired data or by one-way ANOVA. Student's *t*-test for unpaired data is appropriate when only two treatments are to be compared. Use of this test for comparing three or more groups introduces multiple comparisons; e.g., for three treatments, three pair-wise comparisons must be tested (AB, BC, AC). If this approach is used, a correction should be made to assure that the critical level of significance is still $p = 0.05$. The Bonferroni procedure provided such a correction factor.[23]

One-way ANOVA is the usual means of comparing more than two groups for differences. A significant ANOVA can be followed by a post hoc test such as Tukey's or Duncan's to determine where treatment differences lie. Problems of unequal numbers of subjects in treatment groups and unequal variance can have a sizable impact on the outcome of ANOVA in certain situations.[24] Statistical programs such as Statistical Package for the Social Sciences (SPSS) include tests for equality of variances (Bartlett's Box and Cochran's C) as a routine part of the one-way ANOVA output.[19] The results of these tests should be evaluated to determine whether the assumption of homogeneity of variances has been met by the data.

Crossover Design. As the name implies, each subject participates in more than one treatment in crossover design. The advantage of crossover studies is that fewer subjects are required to achieve statistical significance than with parallel design. Each subject is his own control, minimizing variability between treatments. This is accounted for in the ANOVA for a randomized crossover trial, which should include subject, treatment, and phase as main effects.

To demonstrate the advantage of crossover designs, James et al. recently evaluated 59 studies of analgesic efficacy and determined that the variability in data due to subject differences accounted for approximately one-half the residual error.[25] You will recall from the equation used to calculate power that when the error term decreases, power increases. Thus, by using each subject as his own control in a crossover design, the error term can be reduced, and fewer subjects can be utilized to obtain the same precision. For the analgesic efficacy studies, the authors indicated that to obtain the same power, 2.4 times as many subjects would be needed in a parallel study than in a crossover study. When evaluating other drugs, the magnitude of difference in number of subjects needed in the two types of studies will depend on the degree of intersubject variability.[25]

Single-Dose vs. Multiple-Dose vs. Single-Dose/Multiple-Dose. Single-dose studies are, of course, easier to accomplish than multiple-dose studies. Although single-dose studies do not elucidate the true clinical significance of most drug interactions, they do approximate the clinical situation in a few instances.

One instance is when the drugs are only administered together in a single-dose setting. This is exemplified by the interaction of diazepam (used as a premedicant) with ketamine administered during surgery.[26]

A single-dose study also approximates the clinical situation when the effector drug will be administered no more than every fifth half-life. The evaluation of the potential interaction between an antacid and triazolam is essentially equivalent to a steady-state study.

Usually, though, multiple-dose studies provide more definitive data, particularly if conducted in a patient population. They are also the most difficult to accomplish, especially if blinding and crossover procedures are followed. If a multiple-dose interaction study is conducted on an outpatient basis, the investigators lose control of volunteer compliance. Alternatively, conducting the study with subjects in an inpatient facility: (1) requires access to a facility that can handle inpatients for research purposes; (2) makes subject recruitment difficult because of the length of confinement; and (3) increases the cost of conducting the study.

In light of these problems, almost half of the investigators from the 1984 survey chose to evaluate potential drug interactions using a hybrid design: the single-dose/multiple-dose study. This compromise design is an attempt to take advantage of the best aspects of single- and multiple-dose studies. Multiple doses of one drug, usually a potential enzyme inducer or inhibitor, are administered for about five half-lives. A single dose of the second drug, the effector drug, is then administered. All of the cimetidine and ranitidine interaction studies reviewed in the survey were done using this design.

Fastidious vs. Pragmatic. Feinstein has used the classifications fastidious and pragmatic to summarize the controversies in designs of clinical studies. The fastidious design is the most scientifically rigorous, complete with regard to control populations, randomization, blinding, and use of placebos or sham operations. The pragmatic design is the more accomplishable of the two, particularly when working with a patient population as opposed to normal volunteers.[27]

A study of the effect of metoclopramide on absorption of tolfenamic acid in patients with migraine headaches demonstrates the problem of fastidious design. The investigators used a four-way crossover randomized double-blind design. The interaction was evaluated in the subjects in two treatment phases when they were free of migraine, and in two phases within an hour of the onset of a migraine attack. Seven patients completed the four crossover parts of the study.[28] This study design was fastidious, but because of the requirements for enrollment, it took three years to evaluate these seven patients. Thus, the problem of fastidious design in a patient population becomes apparent.

DATA ANALYSIS

When evaluating plasma concentration data, differences in C_{max}, t_{max}, k_e, and AUC are tested using ANOVA. These observations are all univariate and independent and therefore are appropriately evaluated by simple ANOVA. In a drug interaction study, it may also be tempting to compare plasma drug concentrations at individual observation times from the two treatments for differences. Westlake has explained that this is not appropriate because (1) plasma concentration values over time are not independent variables; and (2) comparing many pairs of concentration-time points for differences presents the problem of multiple comparisons.[29]

For significance testing, a p value of 0.05 is often chosen as the minimal critical value. The probability of obtaining at least one significant result in z independent comparisons under the null hypothesis will be $1-(0.95)^z$. Thus, for z = 10 comparisons, the probability is 0.40, i.e., $1-(0.95)^{10}$, that at least one difference will be found by chance alone, not 0.05.[30]

Although this may seem like common knowledge, refereed articles published in respected journals have statements such as: "Plasma concentration data at individual times. . . .were compared for the two formulations by paired t-tests."

Dynamic measurements have the same properties as kinetic assessments. Therefore, they should be given the same statistical considerations. Unfortunately, many reports of multiple comparisons over time using Student's t-test for paired data can be found in the literature.

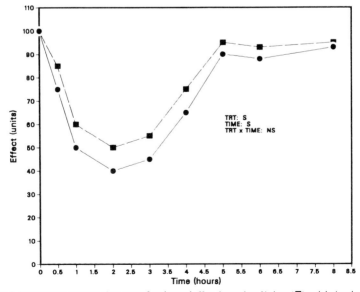

Figue 8. Hypothetical effect vs. time curves for observed effect due to drug X alone (■) and during therapy with drug Y (●). Repeated measures ANOVA would result in significant difference due to treatment (enhanced effect of X during treatment with Y) and time (e.g., overall mean values for effect at time 2 h are different from those at 0 and 4 h).

Analysis of Repeated Assessments. An appropriate means of analyzing data of this type is repeated measures ANOVA, which has been explained in an exceptionally clear fashion by Westlake.[29] For actually performing the analysis, BMDP has an excellent package (program P2V).

In a simple repeated measures analysis model, three factors can be evaluated: the difference due to treatment, the effect of time, and the interaction between treatment and time. The treatment effect is analogous to one-way ANOVA, with the exception that in the one-way procedure, a univariate characteristic is being analyzed. In testing for treatment effect in repeated measures ANOVA, all values for all observation times for the two treatments are compared. To demonstrate the concept, Figure 8 is a plot of hypothetical mean effect data following treatment with drug X (the effector drug) and drugs X + Y. As you can see, the curves are parallel, but the X + Y treatment has a consistently smaller change from baseline. Analysis of the data in this figure by repeated measures ANOVA would result in significant treatment differences.

The evaluation of the time factor is essentially a determination of whether or not mean values for both treatments at any single observation time differ from the mean values at any other time. In this example, there would be a significant time effect. The mean two-hour time observation differs from mean baseline observations.

The ANOVA table for repeated measures design is in two sections, as shown in Table 3. In the first section, there is a test for the differences between the means of the two treatments. As stated, if the treatment F is significant, then there is a statistical difference between therapy with drug X vs. drugs X + Y. The F for time is presented in subplot.

The final F value in the ANOVA table is the interaction term. When this is significant, it denotes that the shapes of the curves for the two treatment groups differ. That is, there are differences between treatments even after they have been adjusted to a mean effect value. An example might be the hypothetical data following drug X and drugs X + Z presented in Figure 9. The means of the effect values for all observation times for X and X + Z are not different; hence, there is

Table 3. Analysis of Variance Table for Repeated Measures*

SOURCE	p VALUE	INTERPRETATION
Mean	S	
Group	S	treatment means differ
Error		
Time	S	effect differs by time
Group-time	S	curve shapes differ
Error		

*Dependent variable: effect observations
S = significant.

no treatment effect. However, the profiles are clearly different, and therefore, the interaction term is significant. To determine where individual differences lie, a post hoc test such as the Student-Newman Keul's can be done using the mean value for each effect-time point from each treatment.

Data Transformation. Often, dynamic data are analyzed in a transformed state, either as normalized data, as percent change from baseline, or as a logarithm. There are some occasions when data transformation is appropriate. However, transforming the data conceals the variability in baseline measurements and alters the distribution of the data. An argument can be offered that perhaps the data do not meet assumptions of normality or equality of variances. Consultation with a statistician and further reading about the failure to meet the assumptions of ANOVA[25] are highly recommended. Unless there is a theoretical basis for transforming the data, analysis should be done on raw data.

Interpretation of Significance Testing. Much has been written about the "significance of significant."[30] Statistical significance does not imply clinical significance. Nor does lack of statistical significance mean that the interaction is not of clinical importance. The actual magnitude of the difference between treatments and the range of observations are important to the interpretation of the data. Recommendations about use and interpretation of statistics from the various editorials on the topic are all similar. Proper statistical evaluation of the data is an impor-

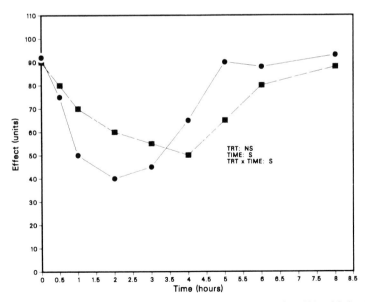

Figure 9. Hypothetical effect vs. time curves for observed effect due to drug X alone (●) and during therapy with drug Z (■). Repeated measures ANOVA results in no difference due to treatments (mean effect values for both treatments for observation times 0-8.25 h are identical). The F values for time and interaction between treatment and time are significant.

tant tool; but as a tool, this evaluation should not inhibit the judgment of the investigators or consumers of the paper. This concept was most succinctly described by *The Inter-Ocular Traumatic Test*: "You know what the data mean when the conclusion hits you between the eyes."[31]

Summary

I would like to share with you the guidelines for conducting a good experiment published in 1958. The requirements for a good drug interaction study are the same as those of any good experiment:

1. Absence from systematic error. This can be accomplished by blinding and randomization procedures.

2. Precision. A good study should have adequate power to detect differences. Steps should be taken to control as many variables as possible and to evaluate the appropriate number of subjects.

3. Range of validity. Can you extrapolate your conclusions to the patient population for whom these drugs will be prescribed?

4. Simplicity of design and analysis. Increasing the complexity of the design increases the likelihood of errors unless very skilled and committed individuals are involved.

5. Proper statistical analysis without artificial assumptions. Analysis of raw data should be the rule unless there is a theoretically sound reason for transforming the data.[32]

References

1. HOLFORD NHG, SHEINER LB. Kinetics of pharmacologic response. *Pharmacol Ther* 1982;*16*:143-66.

2. KOZAK PP, CUMMINS LH, GILLMAN SA. Administration of erythromycin to patients on theophylline. *J Allergy Clin Immunol* 1977;*60*:149-51.

3. PFEIFER HJ, GREENBLATT DJ, FRIEDMAN P. Effects of three antibiotics on theophylline kinetics. *Clin Pharmacol Ther* 1979;*26*:36-40.

4. ZAROWITZ BJM, SZEFLER SJ, LASEZKAY GM. Effect of erythromycin base on theophylline kinetics. *Clin Pharmacol Ther* 1981;*29*:601-5.

5. RENTON KW, GRAY JD, HUNG OR. Depression of theophylline elimination by erythromycin. *Clin Pharmacol Ther* 1981;*30*:422-6.

6. PRINCE RA, WING DS, WEINBERGER MM, HENDELES LS, RIEGELMAN S. Effect of erythromycin on theophylline kinetics. *J Allergy Clin Immunol* 1981;*68*:427-31.

7. MCLEAN AJ, TONKIN A, MCCARTHY P, HARRISON P. Dose dependence of atenolol-ampicillin interaction. *Br J Clin Pharmacol* 1984;*18*:969-70.

8. AGGELER PM, O'REILLY RA, LEONG L, KOWITZ PE. Potentiation of anticoagulant effect of warfarin by phenylbutazone. *N Engl J Med* 1967;*276*:496-501.

9. O'REILLY RA. Studies on the optical enentiomorphs of warfarin in man. *Clin Pharmacol Ther* 1974;*16*:348-54.

10. BANFIELD C, O'REILLY R, CHAN E, ROWLAND M. Phenylbutazone-warfarin interaction in man; further sterochemical and metabolic considerations. *Br J Clin Pharmacol* 1983;*16*:669-75.

11. O'REILLY RA. Dynamic interaction between disulfiram and separated enantiomorphs of racemic warfarin. *Clin Pharmacol Ther* 1981;*29*:332-6.

12. DAS G, BARR CE, CARLSON J. Reduction of digoxin effect during the digoxin-quinidine interaction. *Clin Pharmacol Ther* 1984;*35*:317-21.

13. STOEHR GP, KROBOTH PD, JUHL RP, WENDER DB, PHILLIPS JP, SMITH RB. Effect of oral contraceptives on triazolam, temazepam, alprazolam, and lorazepam kinetics. *Clin Pharmacol Ther* 1984;*36*:683-390.

14. KROBOTH PD, SMITH RB, STOEHR GP, JUHL RP. Pharmacodynamic evaluation of the oral contraceptive-benzodiazepine interaction. *Clin Pharmacol Ther* 1985;*38*:525-32.

15. ELLINWOOD EH, EASLER ME, LINNOILA M, MOLTER DW, HEATHERLY DG, BJORNSSON TD. Effects of oral contraceptives on diazepam-induced psychomotor impairment. *Clin Pharmacol Ther* 1984;*35*:360-6.

16. SMITH RB. Evaluating the effects of disease state and patient variables on pharmacokinetics and pharmacodynamics. In: Smith RB, Kroboth PD, Juhl RP, eds. Pharmacokinetics and pharmacodynamics: research design and analysis. Cincinnati: Harvey Whitney Books, 1986:33-50.

17. FREIMAN JA, CHALMERS TC, SMITH H, KUEBLER RR. The importance of beta, the type II error and sample size in the design and interpretation of the randomized control trial. Survey of 71 "negative" trials. *N Engl J Med* 1978;*299*:690-4.

18. DIXON WJ, MASSEY FJ. Introduction to statistical analysis. 3rd ed. New York: McGraw-Hill Book Company, 1969.

19. WINER BJ. Statistical principles in experimental design. 2nd ed. New York: McGraw-Hill Book Company, 1971.

20. BLAND JM, JONES DR, BENNETT S, COOK DG, HAINES AP, MACFARLANE AJ. Is the clinical trial evidence about new drugs statistically adequate? *Br J Clin Pharmacol* 1985;*19*:155-60.

21. KROBOTH PD, SMITH RB, SILVER MR, et al. The effects of end stage renal disease and aluminum hydroxide on triazolam pharmacokinetics. *Br J Clin Pharmacol* 1985;*19*:839-42.

22. SPILKER B. Guide to clinical studies and developing protocols. New York: Raven Press, 1984.

23. WALLENSTEIN S, ZUCKER CL, FLEISS JF. Some statistical methods useful in circulation research. *Circ Res* 1980;*47*:1-7.

24. GLASS GV, PECKHAM PD, SANDERS JR. Consequences of failure to meet assumptions underlying the fixed effects analyses of variance and covariance. *Rev Educ Res* 1972;*42*:237-88.

25. JAMES KE, FORREST WH, ROSE RL. Crossover and noncrossover designs in four-point parallel line analgesic assays. *Clin Pharmacol Ther* 1985;*37*:242-52.

26. DOMINO EF, DOMINO SE, SMITH RE, et al. Ketamine kinetics in unmedicated and diazepam-premedicated subjects. *Clin Pharmacol Ther* 1984;*36*:645-53.

27. FEINSTEIN A. Presentation at American Society for Clinical Pharmacology and Therapeutics 86th annual meeting, San Antonio, TX. March 28, 1985.

28. TOKOLA RA, NEUVONEN PJ. Effects of migraine attack and metoclopramide on the absorption of tolfenamic acid. *Br J Clin Pharmacol* 1984;*17*:67-75.

29. WESTLAKE WJ. The design and analysis of comparative blood level trials. In: Swarbrick J, ed. Current concepts in the pharmaceutical sciences. Philadelphia: Lea & Febiger, 1973:149-79.

30. Significance of significant. *N Engl J Med* 1968;*278*:1232-3.

31. EDWARDS W, LINDMAN H, SAVAGE LJ. Bayesian statistical inference for psychological research. *Psychol Rev* 1963;*70*:193-242.

32. COX DR. Preliminaries. In: Cox DR, ed. Planning of experiments. New York: John Wiley and Sons, 1958:1-13.

4. EVALUATING THE EFFECTS OF DISEASE STATE AND PATIENT VARIABLES ON PHARMACOKINETICS AND PHARMACODYNAMICS

Randall B. Smith

EVALUATING THE EFFECTS OF DISEASE STATE AND PATIENT VARIABLES ON PHARMACOKINETICS AND PHARMACODYNAMICS

Randall B. Smith

PHARMACOKINETICS has become an important element in the development and utilization of new drug entities as well as in improving the utilization of older drug products. During the developmental years of pharmacokinetic research, studies of a number of drugs demonstrated intersubject variability in absorption, distribution, and elimination that were of sufficient magnitude to alter therapeutic effect. This finding stimulated research in two major areas. The first was the development of clinical pharmacokinetics, in which dosing regimens of drugs such as gentamicin were individualized using plasma concentration-time data. The second was the proliferation of research examining the effects of patients' characteristics (such as age and gender), disease states, and other drugs on the pharmacokinetics of drugs.

The primary assumption in using this information as a basis for dosing recommendations is that there is a direct relationship between drug plasma concentration and drug effect. This concept, however, has been documented to be true and clinically useful for only a few drugs such as phenytoin and theophylline. Actually, the relationship between concentration and effect for most drugs has been poorly understood, making it difficult to extrapolate observed pharmacokinetic changes to clinical significance. The historical lack of sensitive methodologies for determining response to therapeutic agents has contributed to this situation. Now that technology for assaying physiologic fluids for concentrations of many drugs has been developed, there are renewed efforts to develop methods for studying pharmacodynamics in addition to pharmacokinetics. The availability of novel dosage forms has also contributed to the need for pharmacologic response data in selection of appropriate delivery systems.

In this presentation we will consider some of the problems involved in evaluating the influence of patient characteristics and disease states on drug pharmacokinetics and pharmacodynamics. Disease states such as alcoholic liver disease that affect eliminating organ function as well as diseases for which the drugs are used to treat will be examined. The characteristics of the patient population are important considerations in effective design for all studies.

Table 1. Typical Inclusion Criteria for a
Pharmacokinetic Study in Normal Volunteers

Age 21–55 years
Normal screening vital signs
Laboratory parameters within normal range
No history of cardiovascular or other chronic disease
Nonobese (within 15 percent of ideal body weight)
Male
Not taking any chronic medications

Pharmacokinetic Studies

It has been the standard practice to evaluate pharmacokinetics of drug entities in normal populations, controlling as many variables as possible and thus obtaining a reasonably homogeneous population. This practice originated in bioavailability studies where the objective was to evaluate dosage forms with minimal differences among individual subjects. Typical inclusion criteria for these types of studies are found in Table 1.

It is apparent from these criteria that subjects who participate in standard pharmacokinetic studies might provide baseline pharmacokinetic data. However, the data would not necessarily be of use in defining dosage recommendations for patients.

PATIENT CHARACTERISTICS

There are many patient characteristics that have the potential to affect pharmacokinetics and drug response. The most studied of these are age, smoking, obesity, and gender. Less often examined but still of potential importance are factors such as ethnic group, race, and nutritional status. There have been numerous review articles and books that summarize the effects of these patient characteristics on various pharmacokinetic parameters.[1] Our purpose is not to review all of this literature, but rather to explore techniques for determining the pharmacokinetic changes resulting from differences in patient characteristics. Examination of study design to show effects of age and gender will illustrate some potential problems in current methodology.

Age and Gender. Both extremes of the age spectrum present problems in study design. Because of the ethical problems related to informed consent and drug administration with no intended personal benefit, the kinetics of drugs in infants and young children are often determined only during medical therapy. This introduces more uncontrolled variables than if healthy infants or children were studied.

In contrast, studies of the effects of advanced age on pharmacokinetics are usually similar to studies in young healthy subjects. Attempts are made to control as many factors as possible so that age is the only major variable. It is not always easy to recruit elderly subjects who are considered "healthy" in the same sense as normal healthy young subjects. Many of the elderly have compensated chronic disease, history of disease, or are taking medications. Despite this, the general practice is to use healthy elderly subjects even though they may not be representative of the elderly population as a whole.

Effect of sample size. The clinical usefulness of these studies becomes even more questionable in view of the small number of subjects usually evaluated. Figure 1 is a frequency distribution of the number of elderly subjects evaluated in 33 kinetic studies reported in the literature. It is apparent that most of these studies are performed with group sizes of 8 to 10 subjects. The small number of subjects and the variability in pharmacokinetic parameters can make it difficult to make definite recommendations regarding dosage regimens for the elderly. One problem arising from the use of small numbers of subjects can be illustrated by several studies of triazolam in elderly subjects.

The Problem of Conflicting Results. Triazolam (Figure 2) is primarily eliminated from the body by oxidative metabolism to hydroxy metabolites, which undergo rapid conjugation and elimination in urine.[2] Since elderly patients may require short-term therapy for insomnia and since they may have reduced metabolic capacity, it was important to determine if elderly patients cleared triazolam more slowly than young subjects. Two separate studies were performed: study 1 was a single dose in elderly and young subjects,[3] and study 2 was a single-dose crossover comparison of triazolam and temazepam in subjects ranging from 20 to 78 years of age.[4] A summary of the study designs is shown in Table 2.

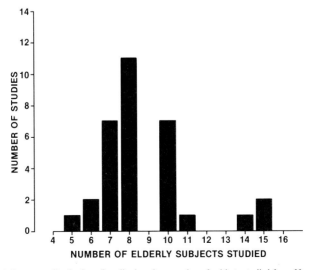

Figure 1. Frequency distribution of studies based on number of subjects studied from 33 published pharmacokinetic studies in elderly.

The results of study 1 showed that triazolam clearance was significantly lower in elderly men and women, but that half-life was not affected. The changes in triazolam clearance with age correlated with the age-related changes in antipyrine clearance ($r = 0.44$). These pharmacokinetic differences suggest that the dose of triazolam should be reduced in elderly patients but that excessive accumulation of drug would not be a problem.[3]

Analysis of kinetic data from study 2 showed no effect of age on either clearance or elimination half-life of triazolam. A significant difference was observed, however, in elimination half-life between elderly men and elderly women. Mean triazolam plasma concentrations for three age groups of men and women are shown in Figure 3. In contrast to study 1, the results of study 2 suggested that the dose reduction is not necessary for triazolam in elderly patients.[4]

Cross-study comparisons are generally invalid because of the differences in data analysis, analytical methodology, protocol procedures, and/or subject populations. In this case, however, the analysis of triazolam plasma concentrations was determined by the same method in the same laboratory, protocol procedures were virtually identical, and the data analysis was performed in the same manner for both studies. Additionally, the mean ages and weights of the groups were almost identical (Table 3).

Table 2. Summary of Study Designs for Two Studies of Triazolam Pharmacokinetics in Elderly

STUDY	SUBJECTS	DOSING
1	1 male, 8 female <35 yr 9 male, 8 female >60 yr	single dose triazolam 0.5 mg po after overnight fast
2	5 male, 5 female 20–39 yr 5 male, 5 female 40–59 yr 5 male, 5 female >60 yr	single dose triazolam 0.5 mg po after overnight fast

Table 3. Comparison of Subject Characteristics for Two Studies of Triazolam Pharmacokinetics in Elderly vs. Young Adults

AGE GROUP	20-39 yr				>60 yr			
GENDER	M		F		M		F	
STUDY	1	2	1	2	1	2	1	2
Number	8	5	8	5	9	5	8	5
Age (yr)	26* (23–33)†	25 (22–28)	25 (21–31)	27 (20–35)	70 (61–78)	72 (68–76)	72 (65–81)	67 (63–71)
Weight (kg)	70 (57–80)	80 (71–89)	57 (48–64)	60 (58–62)	80 (65–96)	77 (56–93)	63 (56–82)	59 (56–71)
Number of Smokers	1	3	0	3	0	0	3	1

*Mean values.

†Numbers in parentheses are ranges.

Examination of the clearance data, however, reveals a possible reason for the differing results. Although clearance of individual elderly subjects in the two studies (Figure 4) were similar, triazolam clearances for the control groups were markedly different.[3,4] Further comparison of the triazolam clearance data with average data from five additional pharmacokinetic studies in normal volunteers (Table 4) suggests that the five control men in study 2 were not representative of the young male population.[5-9]

The difference in clearance between young women in study 1 and those in study 2 was very similar to the difference in clearance we have reported between young women using oral contraceptives and those who were nonusers (Table 4, study 7). Unfortunately, oral contraceptive use was not documented for the female subjects in studies 1 and 2. Thus, this potential explanation for the difference in clearance between the two control populations of women could not be evaluated.

These studies illustrate two problems in evaluating patient characteristics: sample size and selection of the comparison population. These problems are not unique to studies of patient characteristics. They also occur in studies of disease state effects.

DISEASES OF ELIMINATING ORGANS

Although drugs may be eliminated by numerous pathways, the major organs of drug elimination are the liver and kidney. Since diseases of these organs have the potential to dramatically alter the pharmacokinetics of many drugs, it is not surprising that this subject has been a principal focus of clinical pharmacokinetic research. These studies are actually more complex than those concerned with patient characteristics, even though the studies may appear more simple on cursory examination. Selection of a homogeneous group of patients that meets criteria for ''normal'' with the exception of the presence of renal or hepatic disease is difficult. The disease state is an additional parameter to those of age, race, other medications, and so on. Hepatic and renal disease can range from almost normal function to end-stage organ failure. Quantification of the extent of organ failure in the patient population is essential to adequately evaluate effects of organ dysfunction on pharmacokinetics.

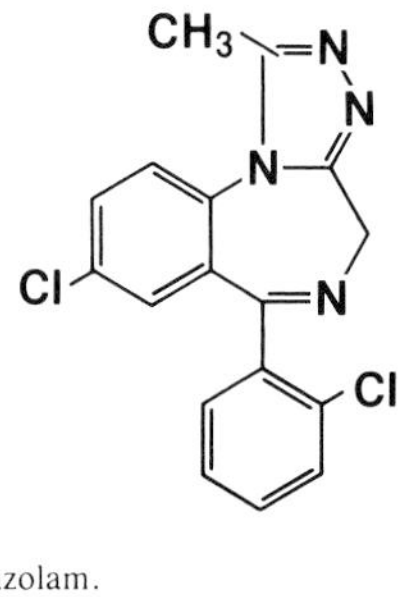

Figure 2. Graphic formula of triazolam.

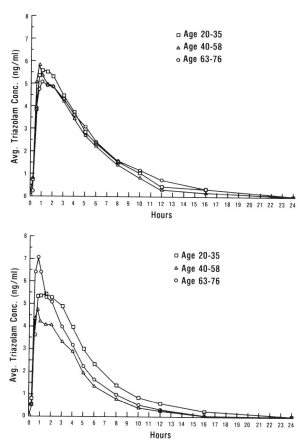

Figure 3. Mean triazolam plasma concentrations after a single oral 0.5 mg dose in three age groups of men (top) and women (bottom) (reproduced with permission from Reference 4).

Table 4. Mean Triazolam Oral Clearance in Young Men and Women from Studies Reported in the Literature

STUDY	MEN (n)	WOMEN (n)	REFERENCE
1	6.2 (8)	8.8 (8)	4
2	3.7 (5)	4.6 (5)	5
3	5.6 (18)		6
4	4.8 (7)		6
5	6.6 (5)		7
6	5.9 (9)		8
7		4.9 (10)*	9
7		7.1 (10)†	9

*Oral contraceptive users.
†No oral contraceptive use.

Renal Disease. The impact of renal disease on drug elimination has been studied more effectively than the effect of hepatic disease. This has resulted from the availability of methods to quantify renal function, the limited reserve of renal function, and the fact that many drugs eliminated in urine are eliminated by mechanistically simple processes, i.e., filtration. Probably the most significant reason for the extensive pharmacokinetic studies in patients with renal disease, however, is the access to patients with renal failure who are maintained on dialysis. These patients provide a relatively homogeneous population with respect to extent of disease. Patients with end-stage renal disease are maintained on either hemodialysis (HD) or continuous ambulatory peritoneal dialysis (CAPD).

HD Patients. Pharmacokinetic studies in HD patients can be designed to evaluate patients on off-dialysis days, during dialysis, or both. Off-dialysis day studies are generally designed to show the change in drug kinetics due to renal failure and to evaluate the potential for drug accumulation. Many of these experiments use single-dose administration of drug on off-dialysis days in 8–10 HD patients compared to a control group of age-, gender-, and weight-matched subjects.

These studies are subject to the same limitations as studies in the elderly because of the small sample size. In addition, the study populations are generally not uniform with respect to patient variables. For example, patient age and gender distribution for five recently published renal disease studies are shown in Table 5.[10-14] Perusal of the literature suggests that the age ranges and sample sizes in these studies are consistent with most renal disease studies. Given the wide range of patient

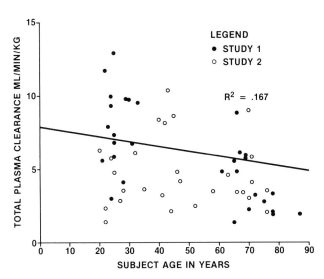

Figure 4. Triazolam oral clearance as a function of age. Combined data from References 3 and 4.

Table 5. Patient Characteristics in Recently Published
Renal Disease Studies

DRUG	NO. OF SUBJECTS		AGE RANGE (yr)	REFERENCE
	MEN	WOMEN		
Cibenzoline	7	7	28–83	10
Temazepam	6	5	18–64	11
Cefotaxime	4	2	50 ± 9.1	12
Cefoperazone	6	1	25–64	13
Lorazepam		(4)	25–53	14

characteristics, it is important to know as much as possible about the influence of these factors on the pharmacokinetics of a drug before developing a protocol to study renal disease.

An appropriate way to control for patient characteristics is to evaluate a large number of patients that would permit stratification by characteristic (e.g., age, weight). Alternatively, when small numbers of patients are evaluated, the ranges of the characteristics should be restricted.

Design Considerations. HD patients studied only on off-dialysis days do not provide complete information for treating patients who will undergo dialysis during therapeutic drug use. Some drug or active metabolites may be removed during dialysis and require replacement. A recent article proposed some guidelines for studies in HD patients. The kinetics of the drug should be determined after intravenous administration, if possible, on a nondialysis day. If the drug has a sufficiently long half-life, drug concentrations should be determined during and after dialysis. For a short half-life drug, intravenous administration should be repeated on a dialysis day with the dialysis procedure performed after drug distribution is complete. Gibson also recommends methods for determining the amount of drug removed during dialysis and calculating replacement doses.[15] While these are reasonable guidelines, additional information would be desirable when considering drugs commonly prescribed for HD patients. Studies evaluating drug and metabolite accumulation and dialysis clearance after multiple doses provide the most clinically useful pharmacokinetic data.

Evaluation of Metabolites. Most studies concerning the effect of renal disease on drugs that undergo some degree of hepatic metabolism rarely determine the effect on disposition of metabolites. This is a major deficiency since metabolites of many compounds are eliminated in urine as unchanged metabolites or as conjugates. These processes may be altered even though metabolism of the parent compound is little affected by renal failure. If the metabolites are pharmacologically active, the importance of determining their kinetic changes is obvious. Determining metabolite kinetics may also be important when the metabolites are inactive, as in the case of lorazepam glucuronide pharmacokinetics. Lorazepam is eliminated by glucuronide conjugation; renal disease has been reported not to affect the elimination of lorazepam.[16] Verbeeck and coworkers, however, reported a kinetic study in two patients with end-stage renal disease who, after multiple doses of drug, showed a dramatic increase in lorazepam elimination half-life. This was postulated to result from the excessive accumulation of the glucuronide metabolite and its hydrolysis back to lorazepam.[17] Lorazepam kinetics in renal disease were subsequently studied after single and multiple doses in six patients with renal impairment and four patients on dialysis. The prolonged lorazepam half-life, observed after both single and multiple doses, was apparently due to an increase in the volume of distribution without a change in clearance.[14] These lorazepam studies demonstrate the importance of evaluating effects of disease states on metabolites as well as parent compounds and show that multiple-dose studies may be necessary.

Patients with Compromised Renal Function. Since end-stage disease represents only a small portion of the renal disease patient population, it is important that drugs be evaluated in patients with varying degrees of renal function. Fortunately, the relationship between degrees of renal insufficiency and changes in pharmacokinetics can be determined using creatinine clearance as a measure of renal function. These studies require utilization of a large number of patients spread over the entire range of renal function. This permits regression analysis of drug clearance as a function of the continuous variable creatinine clearance. A strong correlation between creatinine clearance and drug renal clearance has been demonstrated for a number of drugs, which permits one to estimate the renal clearance of a drug and thus an appropriate dosing regimen for a patient with renal disease.[18]

Hepatic Disease. The effect of hepatic disease on pharmacokinetics is evaluated in much the same manner as the effects of age and renal failure. Hepatic disease studies are more difficult to interpret because of the many etiologies of hepatic dysfunction and the variable effects of disease on metabolic capacity. The extent of metabolic dysfunction is also less easily quantified. There are many enzyme systems in the liver that metabolize drugs and these systems may be affected differently by hepatic disease. It would be almost impossible to find a single endogenous or exogenous substance that could serve as a universal marker of metabolic capacity. However, antipyrine and indocyanine green have found acceptance as metabolic markers of hepatic function.

Antipyrine. Antipyrine is oxidatively metabolized by the P-450 enzyme system and has been used as a marker of oxidative metabolism in many clinical pharmacokinetic studies. Antipyrine elimination half-lives determined in patients with hepatic diseases of different etiologies were recently reported by Narang et al. Average antipyrine elimination half-life was prolonged in all of the disease states. There was considerable intersubject variability, however, and some patients had antipyrine elimination half-lives within the normal range.[19]

Indocyanine Green. Indocyanine green clearance from the body is limited primarily by blood flow to the liver. Although indocyanine green and antipyrine are eliminated differently by the liver, the distinction may not be important in quantifying effects of hepatic disease on metabolic function. There appears to be a relationship between metabolic capacity and blood flow to the liver in chronic liver disease. As Branch et al. have shown, there is a correlation between antipyrine clearance and indocyanine green clearance.[20] This result suggests that for patients with chronic disease, either compound can be used to classify the extent of liver dysfunction.

Importance of Metabolic Markers. The importance of using a marker of hepatic function in pharmacokinetic studies in liver disease patients can be illustrated by a study of the effect of alcoholic liver disease on the kinetics of ibuprofen and sulindac. Fifteen patients with biopsy-confirmed alcoholic liver disease but without ascites, renal disease, or active cardiac disease were recruited for the study. Indocyanine green clearance was determined in all subjects as a measure of hepatic function. Even though the patients seemed categorically similar, the results of the indocyanine green tests indicated there were two subsets of patients in the group. Some patients had an almost normal indocyanine green half-life, while others had a significantly prolonged indocyanine green half-life. The patients were arbitrarily divided into two groups for analysis; nine patients whose indocyanine green half-lives were < 10 minutes (mean = 5.0 minutes) and six patients with indocyanine green half-lives > 10 minutes (mean = 18.3 minutes).[21] Had the indocyanine green data not been available and subjects with indocyanine green half-lives of < 10 minutes been recruited by chance, a study would have been conducted in patients with documented cirrhosis but almost normal drug metabolizing capacity. Results from these patients would have shown little change in drug kinetics and could lead to the erroneous conclusion that there was no need to adjust dosage in hepatic disease. By grouping the patients according to indocyanine green half-life, a correlation between dye clearance and the absorption rate of sulindac and the formation and elimination of sulindac metabolites was demonstrated.

As in studies of kinetics in renal disease patients, hepatic disease study populations are generally small and include patients with a substantial range of age. Therefore, the previously discussed caveats for studies in the elderly and in patients with renal disease apply for studies in hepatic disease.

SELECTION OF THE CONTROL GROUP

Because of the range of ages of subjects evaluated in renal, hepatic, or other disease state studies, the practice of including age-, weight-, and gender-matched control subjects for comparison is generally accepted as necessary. However, the elderly studies previously cited demonstrate that intersubject variability can occur even in the control group and can affect the conclusions of the study. Thus, matching control subjects for age may be of limited value when small numbers of subjects are used. Other factors such as diet, concomitant drug use, and smoking may equally contribute to the variability in kinetics of a given drug, and the control population is rarely matched for these characteristics. A potential value of the control group is to show that assay methods and parameter estimation techniques employed give results comparable to previously reported literature values for a similar population. A control group used for this purpose need not be identically matched to the disease group, and in fact may actually be more useful if it is representative of normal populations cited in the literature.

OTHER CONSIDERATIONS

The evaluation of pharmacokinetics in the elderly using this classic single-dose study design often yields results that are difficult to apply to therapy. Although the studies cited were conducted in the elderly, a single-dose pharmacokinetic study still leaves important questions unanswered. Is a change in drug concentration important in terms of side effects and therapy? Do the elderly exhibit diurnal variation in absorption and/or elimination of the drug? Do active metabolites accumulate? Does the drug exhibit dose-dependent pharmacokinetics?

Presently, there is a common approach to the evaluation of the effects of patient characteristics, renal disease, and hepatic disease on drug disposition. These types of studies all have value in that they can indicate potential problems with the drug in these populations. They also can provide a mechanistic rationale for the observed changes in kinetics. Therefore, these studies need to be done and should include, where appropriate, determination of plasma protein binding, plasma concentrations of metabolites in addition to unchanged drug, clearance of a metabolic marker, and sufficient plasma samples to determine clearance, elimination half-life, and volume of distribution. These studies should also include a dosage range to detect dose dependency in kinetic parameters.

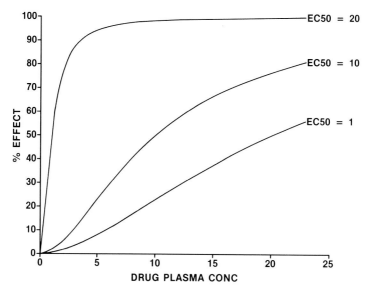

Figure 5. Simulated effect-plasma concentration curves using Equation 1 and varying the constant for the concentration that gives 50 percent of maximal response.

Pharmacodynamic Studies

The studies described above may provide excellent pharmacokinetic information but would not permit any definitive conclusion about clinical relevance. Changes in pharmacokinetics may or may not lead to a change in pharmacologic response, which depends upon the plasma concentration-response relationship. A typical plasma concentration-effect curve can be described by the E_{max} model:

$$E = E_{max} \bullet C^s / (EC_{50}{}^s + C^s) \qquad \text{(Eq. 1)}$$

where E = observed effect, E_{max} = maximum effect, EC_{50} = concentration that gives 50 percent of the maximum response, C = plasma concentration, and s = constant.[22] This equation results in effect-concentration curves illustrated in Figure 5. In order to evaluate possible consequences of reduced renal or hepatic clearance on drug effects, a series of simulations were done using this model.

PHARMACOKINETIC CHANGES

When drug plasma concentrations increase from reduced clearance, an increase in drug effect would be predicted. This is illustrated by the simulation results in Figures 6a and 6b. However, if normal doses of a drug result in plasma concentrations much higher than that which produces 50 percent of the maximal response, increases in drug plasma concentrations will result in little additional effect. This is illustrated in Figure 6c, which demonstrates that despite the 30 percent decrease in clearance, little change in effect results. Changes in drug concentrations due to changes in clearance will result in the largest changes in effect when plasma concentrations are in the range that produces 20–80 percent response.

PHARMACODYNAMIC CHANGES

Changes in response may occur, however, with only minimal changes in drug plasma concentrations. There are numerous reports of increased drug sensitivity in elderly patients[23] and patients with renal[24] or hepatic disease.[25,26] If a disease state alters the interaction of drug with the receptor, the number of receptors, or the intensity of the response to the drug-receptor interaction, significant changes in observed drug response can occur in spite of limited influence of the disease state on pharmacokinetic parameters. The effect of changes in sensitivity to the drug without a change in pharmacokinetics is illustrated in Figure 3. At a given plasma concentration the responses are markedly different on the three curves that were calculated using the same E_{max} value but different EC_{50} values. Thus, studies demonstrating that a disease state does not alter pharmacokinetic parameters do not provide adequate evidence that a drug could be given at normal doses in that particular patient population.

DESIGN REQUIREMENTS

A logical approach to lending clinical validity to a pharmacokinetic study is to measure drug response in addition to the pharmacokinetic parameters determined in the study. This could range from simple assessment of one pharmacologic parameter a few times to assessing many responses at frequent intervals. No matter how simple the measurements to be made, the introduction of pharmacologic measurements to a pharmacokinetic trial causes major change to the design and logistics of the trial.

Factors such as blinding and placebo comparisons, which may not have been important in a pharmacokinetic study, become extremely important in determining the validity of pharmacodynamic measurements.

Blinding and Placebo Comparisons. Blinding the person conducting the trial is not necessary in a pharmacokinetic study since the observer has no effect on drug plasma concentrations. For most pharmacologic measurements, however, bias may be introduced by the investigator and/or the person making the assessments. Subjects can also bias their response, particularly with measurements that require cooper-

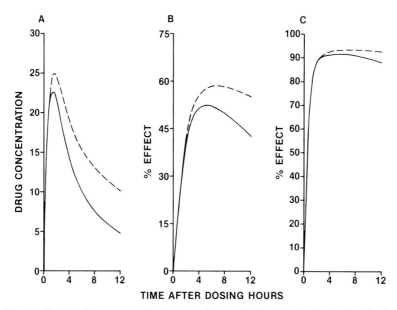

Figure 6a. Simulated plasma concentration-time curves for normal subjects (——) and renal or hepatic subjects (-----) with a 30 percent reduction in clearance.

b. Calculated response curves based on plasma concentrations in (A) when EC_{50} is similar to average plasma concentration.

c. Calculated response curves based on plasma concentrations in (A) when EC_{50} is much lower than the average plasma concentration.

ation. Thus, both the investigators and subjects should be blinded in pharmacodynamic trials to avoid bias. Pharmacologic response to the drug must also be tested in comparison to response to placebo. Even the most simple pharmacodynamic study should be designed as a double-blind, placebo-controlled, randomized study. This adds to the difficulty of conducting the study. Making pharmacologic measurements also may require access to sophisticated equipment and require additional personnel. The open-label drug supplies used for a pharmacokinetic study must be replaced by blinded supplies with matching placebo dosage forms; this causes a time delay. These factors add not only to the complexity of the study, but also to the cost.

Exclusion Criteria. Patient recruitment for pharmacodynamic studies may be difficult because of additional exclusion criteria. As an example, Parker and Roberts described recruitment of hepatic disease patients for a pharmacodynamic study as follows:

"...when studying both the metabolism and the action of a central nervous system depressant in patients with hepatic cirrhosis it is necessary to adopt a number of stringent exclusion criteria. In this study exclusion of patients who had been encephalopathic, or who were taking enzyme inducers such as anticonvulsants or inhibitors such as cimetidine and those on centrally acting drugs hampered recruitment in the study. Thus it took a full year to recruit nine patients...."[26]

Study Design. Study conditions and/or procedures may alter the pharmacologic response. For example, obtaining the blood sample may affect the sedation of a subject. Therefore, the appropriate order of obtaining pharmacologic measurements and blood samples must be determined. Diurnal variation in pharmacologic effects is often pronounced due to physiologic changes in the sleep-wake cycle. Tolerance can develop to some of the pharmacologic effects of drugs. A single-dose evaluation may lead to a different interpretation of the clinical importance than would result from a multiple-dose study. It is also important that either a single dose sufficient to cause a measurable effect or a range of doses be administered.

ALTERNATIVE APPROACHES

Diseases of the liver and kidney are not the only disease states that have the potential to alter the pharmacokinetics and/or pharmacodynamics of a drug. The disposition and response to a drug should be determined in those patients the drug is used to treat. There are several approaches that may be employed to obtain this data.

Intensive Sampling Design. One method of studying a drug during therapeutic use would be to design a study similar to the pharmacokinetic and pharmacodynamic trials we have described. Instead of normal volunteers the subjects would be patients who need the drug for treatment. Patients would be administered drug according to their normal dosing regimen, with the patient confined on selected days for intensive blood sampling and evaluation. Such a study could provide excellent data, although the cost would be prohibitive and only a small number of patients could be studied this intensively. The small number of subjects would then make it difficult to extrapolate the results to the general patient population.

Limited Sampling Design. An alternative approach for studying drug during therapeutic use would be to evaluate a larger number of patients, but obtain fewer blood samples. This strategy presents certain problems in evaluating the data since we have limited samples for each patient. This usually involves obtaining plasma concentrations at the same times in all patients, i.e., nadir values. The mean data are then compared with response. This type of analysis is often subject to significant error due to variation in the timing of blood samples relative to dose administration and to variability in intervals between doses, regardless of the directions in the protocol. It is also rarely possible to derive meaningful parameters from these data and especially difficult to relate these levels to therapeutic response or to side effects. Should accurate records be kept regarding the times of dosing and blood sampling, it would be possible to analyze the pooled data by conventional nonlinear regression techniques. An even better approach would be to design studies allowing samples to be obtained at any time or within certain time ranges to be collected. This would require accurate documentation of dose and time of blood sampling. These data would then be amenable to population kinetic analysis, which permits evaluation of patient population subsets stratified by age, gender, or other characteristics. This analysis is discussed in detail by Grasela elsewhere in this symposium (pages 85–103).

As in the case of hepatic and renal studies, it is important that pharmacologic responses are evaluated in studies of disease effects. Both approaches we have discussed, i.e., small number of subjects-intensive sampling (classical) or large number of subjects-limited sampling (population), have importance in pharmacodynamic evaluation. The intensive sampling design generally permits a better evaluation of the time course of effects for sophisticated measurements that would be too costly to include in a large-scale study. Also, a number of different measurements can be made in these studies and evaluated to determine which of them would be most valuable to include and to select appropriate times to sample in a limited sampling design study. The results can provide an indication of the variability of the measurements in a well controlled setting. Because large numbers of subjects can be evaluated, the limited sampling design study is the most appropriate for determining the relationship between clinical outcome and drug plasma concentrations.

Summary

Clinical pharmacokinetic studies have been useful in establishing clinically relevant dosing guidelines for only a few drugs. For these drugs, the relationship between clinical outcome and steady-state drug plasma concentrations has been established. This relationship has not been determined for the majority of drugs, yet results from pharmacokinetic studies have been used as the basis for recommending changes in dosing regimens. Although useful for providing an indication of potential therapeutic problems, these studies rarely permit a conclusion about the clinical relevance of observed changes in plasma concentration. A positive trend in research has been to incorporate pharmacodynamic measurements in classical kinetic studies to permit a determination of the clinical relevance of observed changes in kinetics. The addition of pharmacodynamic measurements to a kinetic study, however, requires changes in study design.

Just as advances in analytical methodology made pharmacokinetic studies feasible, research into better methods of measuring pharmacologic effects will result in greater ability to determine pharmacodynamics. There is also an increasing awareness that the data base from intensive studies in small numbers of patients is not adequate to recommend dosing guidelines and that data from a much larger number of patients (i.e., population studies) is required. It seems clear that both types of studies, classical and population designs, are necessary and useful in understanding drug pharmacodynamics. Future research should be focused on developing better pharmacologic measurements and applying those techniques to the evaluation of response changes due to pharmacokinetics and/or disease states.

References

1. GIBALDI M, PRESCOTT L, eds. Handbook of clinical pharmacokinetics. New York: ADIS Health Science Press, 1983.
2. EBERTS FS, PHILOPOULOS Y, REINKE LM, VLIEK RW. Triazolam disposition. *Clin Pharmacol Ther* 1981;*29*:81-93.
3. GREENBLATT DJ, DIVOLL M, ABERNETHY DR, MOSCHITTO LJ, SMITH RB, SHADER RI. Reduced clearance of triazolam in old age: relation to antipyrine oxidizing capacity. *Br J Clin Pharmacol* 1983;*15*:303-9.
4. SMITH RB, DIVOLL M, GILLESPIE WR, GREENBLATT DJ. Effect of subject age and gender on the pharmacokinetics of oral triazolam and temazepam. *J Clin Psychopharmacol* 1983;*3*:172-6.
5. DEHLIN O, BJORNSON G, BJORNSON L, ABRAHAMSSON L, SMITH RB. Pharmacokinetics of triazolam in geriatric patients. *Eur J Clin Pharmacol* 1983;*25*:91-4.
6. Data on file. Kalamazoo, MI: The Upjohn Company.
7. OCHS HR, GREENBLATT DJ, ARENDT RM. Pharmacokinetic noninteraction of triazolam and ethanol. *J Clin Psychopharmacol* 1984;*4*:106-7.
8. ABERNETHY DR, GREENBLATT DG, DIVOLL M, SHADER RI. Interaction of cimetidine with the triazolobenzodiazepines alprazolam and triazolam. *Psychopharmacology* 1983;*80*:275-8.
9. STOEHR GP, KROBOTH PD, JUHL RP, WENDER DB, PHILLIPS JP, SMITH RB. Effect of oral contraceptives on triazolam, temazepam, alprazolam, and lorazepam kinetics. *Clin Pharmacol Ther* 1984;*36*:683-90.
10. CANAL M, FLOUVAT B, AUBERT P, GUEDON J, PRINSEAU J, GABLIN A. Pharmacokinetics of cibenzoline in patients with renal impairment. *J Clin Pharmacol* 1985;*25*:197-203.

11. KROBOTH PD, SMITH RB, RAULT R, et al. Effects of end-stage renal disease and aluminum hydroxide on temazepam kinetics. *Clin Pharmacol Ther* 1985;*37*:454-9.

12. KAMPF D, BORNER K, MOLLER M, KESSEL M. Kinetic interactions between azlocillin, cefotaxime, and cefotaxime metabolites in normal and impaired renal function. *Clin Pharmacol Ther* 1984;*35*:214-20.

13. KELLER E, JANSEN A, KLAUS P, HOPPE-SEYLER G, SCHOLLMEYER P. Intraperitoneal and intravenous cefoperazone kinetics during continuous ambulatory peritoneal dialysis. *Clin Pharmacol Ther* 1984;*35*:208-13.

14. MORRISON G, CHIANG ST, KOEPKE HH, WALKER BR. Effect of renal impairment and hemodialysis on lorazepam kinetics. *Clin Pharmacol Ther* 1984;*35*:646-52.

15. GIBSON TP. Problems in designing hemodialysis drug studies. *Pharmacotherapy* 1985;*5*:23-9.

16. MEYER BR. Benzodiazepines in the elderly. *Med Clin North Am* 1982;*66*:1017-35.

17. VERBEECK RK, TJANDRAMAGA TB, DE SCHEPPER PJ, VERBERCKMOES R. Impaired elimination of lorazepam following subchronic administration in two patients with renal failure. *Br J Clin Pharmacol* 1981;*12*:749-51.

18. KEYS PW. Digoxin. In: Evans WE, Schentag JJ, Jusko WJ, eds. Applied pharmacokinetics. San Francisco: Applied Therapeutics, Inc., 1980:334-40.

19. NARANG APS, DATTA DV, MATHUR VS. In vitro drug metabolism in humans with different liver diseases. *Int J Clin Pharmacol Ther Tox* 1983;*21*:496-8.

20. BRANCH RA, HERBERT CM, READ AE. Determinants of serum antipyrine half-lives in patients with liver disease. *Gut* 1973;*14*:569-73.

21. JUHL RP, VAN THIEL DH, DITTERT LW, ALBERT KS, SMITH RB. Ibuprofen and sulindac kinetics in alcoholic liver disease. *Clin Pharmacol Ther* 1983;*34*:104-9.

22. HOLFORD NHG, SHEINER LB. Kinetics of pharmacologic response. *Pharmacol Ther* 1982;*16*:143-66.

23. MEYER BR. Benzodiazepines in the elderly. *Med Clin North Am* 1982;*66*:1017-35.

24. DUNDEE JW, RICHARDS RK. Effect of azotemia upon the action of intravenous barbiturate anesthesia. *Anesthesiology* 1954;*15*:333-46.

25. BRANCH RA, MORGAN MH, JAMES J, READ AE. Intravenous administration of diazepam in patients with chronic liver disease. *Gut* 1976;*17*:975-83.

26. PARKER G, ROBERTS CJC. Plasma concentrations and central nervous system effects of the new hypnotic agent zopiclone in patients with chronic liver disease. *Br J Clin Pharmacol* 1983;*16*:259-65.

5. DRUG EFFECT DETERMINATION: PROVEN AND POTENTIAL METHODOLOGIES

Randall J. Erb

Pharmacological Response
  Dose-Response Relationship
  Effect-Concentration Relationship
    Linear kinetics
    Nonlinear kinetics
    Active metabolites

Variability in Response

Selection of a Pharmacologic Response
  Pilot Studies
  Design Considerations
    Subject acclimation
    Placebo control

Example Uses of Pharmacologic Response
  Digital Plethysmography
    Methodology
    Application to nitroglycerin
  Prolactin Elevation Response
    Methodology
    Application to perphenazine
  Spectral Edge Analysis of Electroencephalography
    Methodology
    Application to alprazolam
  Infrared Thermography
    Methodology
    Applications
Summary

DRUG EFFECT DETERMINATION: PROVEN AND POTENTIAL METHODOLOGIES

Randall J. Erb

IN RECENT YEARS, biopharmaceutics and pharmacokinetics have taken on a significant role in new drug development and evaluation. The establishment of bioequivalence of formulations has become extremely important to the pharmaceutical industry. The purpose of this article is to elucidate the use of pharmacological response variables for evaluating drug product formulations for their bioavailability or clinical attributes.

The Code of Federal Regulations defines bioavailability as the rate and extent to which the active drug ingredient or therapeutic moiety is absorbed from a drug product and becomes available at the site of action.[1] As a practical matter, this definition generally refers to the amount of drug measured in the bloodstream, which may or may not be closely associated with the site of action. Bioavailability might more aptly be defined as the rate and extent of absorption of an active drug moiety into a biological compartment from which a quantitative measurement of drug presence can be made.

The most relevant biological compartment for the measurement of bioavailability for scientific or regulatory purposes depends on the drug in question and the state-of-the-art for making accurate assay measurements or pharmacological response determinations. This is recognized in the regulations, which state that bioavailability determinations can be made by chemical assay of biological fluids, measurement of an acute pharmacological response, or clinical end point evaluations.[1]

Pharmacological Response

A pharmacological response is any measurable physiological response directly attributable to the presence of drug. It may or may not be a therapeutic response of the drug. In order to be useful as a quantitative tool for measuring drug bioavailability, however, several criteria should be met.

A pharmacological response to a drug should be monotonically increasing. As the drug concentration increases in the biological compartment, the response should continuously increase. If, as can occasionally happen, an increase in drug causes a reversal of direction in pharmacological response, the usefulness of the pharmacological response as a quantitative tool becomes limited.

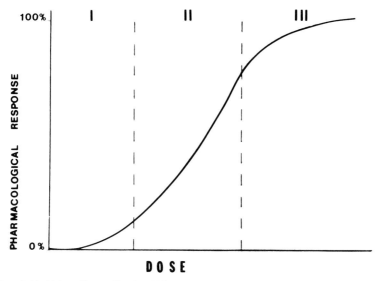

Figure 1. Model dose-effect profile; sigmoidal curve.

DOSE-RESPONSE RELATIONSHIP

Classically, one would expect a dose-response curve to be sigmoidal in nature. A certain minimum amount of drug is needed in the biophase before a pharmacological response can be quantitated (area I of Figure 1). The most useful pharmacological responses will approximate dose-effect curve linearity over the therapeutic range. This is represented by area II of Figure 1. When the amount of drug in the biophase becomes too high, the pharmacological response becomes saturated (area III of Figure 1). Here an increase in drug concentration will cause little or no increase in response.

Optimally, a pharmacological response to a drug should be linear over the range of dose evaluation. A unit of drug increase will cause a proportionate increase in response. Nonlinear relationships can be handled, but a linear relationship means that a pharmacological response unit can be considered a direct measure of relative bioavailability without correction.

To be most useful, a quantitative pharmacological response should occur within the therapeutic dose range of the drug. Little use can be made of a response that is so sensitive it saturates at low doses or a response that requires doses of the drug beyond the therapeutic range to achieve sensitivity.

EFFECT-CONCENTRATION RELATIONSHIP

Perhaps the most misunderstood points concerning the usefulness of pharmacological data revolve around the relationship between drug blood levels and therapeutic activity. No direct correlation with blood levels or therapeutic response is necessary for a pharmacological response to be useful for evaluating drug formulations. Let us see why this is the case.

Linear Kinetics. Given that linear kinetics hold for the system over the therapeutic dose range, the intensity of the physiological response in the therapeutic and pharmacological response compartments (I_t and I_p, respectively) can be described by generalized multiexponential equations as shown in Figure 2. The concentration of drug in the blood can be similarly described by such an equation. Although curve parameters such as I_{max}, C_{max}, t_{max}, and the area under the curve (AUC) may be different in each compartment, as one changes the dose (D) delivered to the system, linearity dictates that I_{max}, C_{max}, and AUC must change by the same proportion in each compartment. Therefore, in studies that compare drug formulations for bioequivalence, it makes no difference which compartment is sampled for the bioavailability data to obtain a valid comparison between dosage forms (assuming similar variation in the data of the compartments, of course).

Nonlinear Kinetics. Drugs that have dose-dependent kinetics can also be tested for bioequivalence because the pharmacological response profiles of formulations that deliver drug similarly must produce the same pharmacological profile. One must be cautioned about drawing any conclusions regarding dose proportionality for formulations that do not produce the same pharmacological profile, however.

Active Metabolites. One of the elements of using pharmacological response that seems to cause confusion is the role of active metabolites. In the case where the study is a bioequivalence study, active metabolites are not really a problem. In fact, this situation is analogous to using a nonspecific assay to determine bioequivalence of two dosage forms. The point is, if two dosage forms are in theory delivering drug at the same rate and extent, the pharmacological profiles of the dosage forms must be identical. To go one step further, if a pharmacological response is linearly dose-dependent and the dosage form is an immediate release dosage form, then the percent difference in the pharmacological response is identical to the percent difference between the strengths of the dosage forms tested. This is predetermined by the

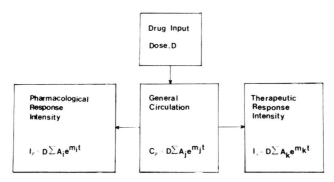

Figure 2. Conceptualized linear compartment model relating a pharmacological response with therapeutic response and drug in circulation. Linearity allows sampling of any of these compartments to determine relative bioavailability (bioequivalence).

relationship between drug input and pharmacological output, which has a unique mathematical solution.

In the situation where controlled-release dosage forms are being tested for bioequivalence, any difference in rate or extent of delivery confounds results in such a way that no absolute information is available concerning bioavailability. On the other hand, if the pharmacological profiles are identical for two dosage forms, their rate and extent of delivery must be identical.

Variability In Response

Variation in data derived to evaluate drug product bioavailability or clinical efficacy is of utmost importance. Sources of variation include dosage form delivery rate, absorption, distribution, metabolism, excretion, and receptor site sensitivity changes. The accuracy with which one can measure the cumulative effect of these variations depends in part on the sensitivity of the biological fluid assay or pharmacological response.

Although it is tacitly assumed that pharmacological response data are more variable than blood level data, this is not necessarily the case. Data generated by this author demonstrates that in some instances pharmacological data variation is actually smaller than variation in blood level data. For instance, small sample statistical calculations have demonstrated that pupillometry (change in the size of the pupil of the eye) can detect a 25 percent difference in 100 mg doses of thioridazine (alpha = 0.05, beta = 0.01) using only 17 subjects. Digital plethysmography (DPG) requires 30 subjects to detect a 25 percent difference between isosorbide dinitrate 40 mg controlled release products (alpha = 0.05, beta = 0.20). Using phenothiazine-induced prolactin response, a 20 percent difference can be detected in trifluoperazine 5 mg po and perphenazine 16 mg using 32 and 24 subjects, respectively (alpha = 0.05, beta = 0.20). The power in these statistics is comparable to that found using blood levels, and, in some cases, it is superior.

Selection Of A Pharmacologic Response

Whether or not a pharmacological response is practical for use in drug testing depends on both regulatory and scientific considerations. It will depend on whether biological assay methodologies exist, and whether it is feasible to measure an appropriate pharmacological response. If biological fluid assays are nonexistent, certainly a pharmacological response approach may be the only option. If chemical assay methods do exist, whether a pharmacological approach is justified will depend on its sensitivity and reliability compared to the existing assay method. Federal regulations contain a built-in bias presupposing that any existing chemical assay method is always preferable to a pharmacological method. Before using any pharmacological approach, it is always best to have the protocol approved by the Food and Drug Administration.

PILOT STUDIES

From the scientific aspect, one must determine whether the drug in question reliably produces a measurable, dose-dependent, monotonically increasing, and (hopefully) linear response in human volunteers taking doses in the therapeutic range.

To find out, a pilot study using a small number of healthy male subjects should be conducted. The author has found that four to six subjects administered a placebo dose and three doses of drug (distributed within the normal therapeutic range) in a double-blind crossover experiment provides a good pilot study to determine whether a particular pharmacological response is viable. Experience has shown that if a response is going to be practical, dose-dependent trends will be obvious in this small study. In nearly every case where a pharmacological response was eventually determined to be useful, dose levels were statistically significantly different (alpha = 0.05) from each other by analysis of variance using four to six subjects.

DESIGN CONSIDERATIONS

Subject Acclimation. Pharmacological responses are most often calculated as a percent change from predrug activity. Test subjects must be allowed to adjust to the experimental environment in order to normalize their physiological baseline. Before the study begins, it is best to conduct a screening run with a small dose of the drug to acclimate subjects to the experimental conditions. During the actual run day, it is a good practice to ignore the first and last data taken to determine the average predrug baseline. This will minimize data artifacts due to initial adjustment to the experimental conditions.

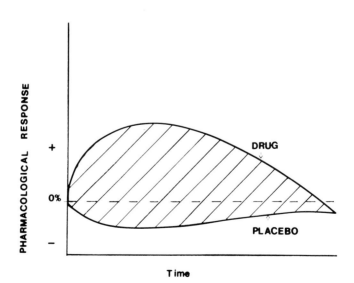

Figure 3. Drug activity (crosshatched area) is represented by the difference between the drug response curve (top) and the placebo response curve (bottom).

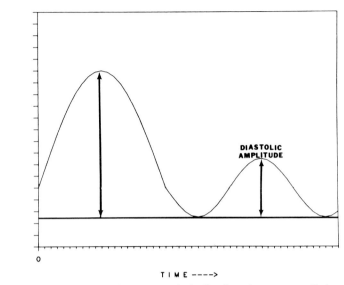

Figure 4. The digital plethysmographic waveform. Increases in the diastolic peak represent vasodilation.

Placebo Control. It is very important to incorporate a placebo dose into pharmacological response studies in order to establish baseline data. All comparisons of activity of the doses should be made on the basis of placebo-corrected activity of the dose, not on the absolute activity of the dose. To see the significance of this, refer to Figure 3, which shows a hypothetical activity profile of a drug over time compared to placebo. The magnitude of activity of the drug is represented by the crosshatched area. This is the placebo-corrected response of the drug. Only in the case where a placebo dose has no effect on the baseline response is the drug response the absolute change in pharmacological response.

Example Uses Of Pharmacologic Response

Functional pharmacological responses include simple measurements such as blood pressure, size of the pupil of the eye, or blood hormone levels. They can also be rather obtuse calculated parameters extracted from complex physiological signals such as the electrocardiogram or electroencephalogram (EEG). For example, DPG has demonstrated a linear dose-dependent response for oral controlled-release nitroglycerin and has been used in > 100 studies to evaluate the bioavailability characteristics of other peripheral vasodilators.[2-5] The rise in prolactin has been used to quantitate phenothiazine bioavailability. Spectral edge analysis of EEG has been employed to evaluate the temporal effects of alprazolam on brain function. Computerized electronic thermography has been used to evaluate the vasodilatory effect of beta-blockers[6] and the antiinflammatory effect of antiinflammatory drugs (data on file, R.J. Erb, 1985).

DIGITAL PLETHYSMOGRAPHY

Methodology. Detecting blood levels of vasodilator drugs is extremely difficult, if not impossible. In 1977 the FDA published a guideline recommending the use of DPG for the bioavailability determination of peripheral vasodilators.[2] Since then the author has conducted >100 studies using DPG that have evaluated various delivery systems containing nitroglycerin,[7,8] isosorbide dinitrate, pentaerythritol tetranitrate, and erythrityl tetranitrate.[5]

The DPG methodology uses the waveform of the blood pressure pulse that occurs at the tip of the finger to determine the relative state of vasodilation of the circulatory system. DPG waveform (Figure 4) changes are relatively straightforward to analyze, sensitive to very low doses of nitroglycerin, and clinically relevant.

As vasodilators become available to the bloodstream, they cause venous and arterial dilation. This dilation produces a change in the DPG diastolic peak amplitude of the waveform (Figure 4). The amplitude of the diastolic portion of the waveform depends upon the amount of fluid wave rebound of blood bouncing off the aortic valve as it closes.

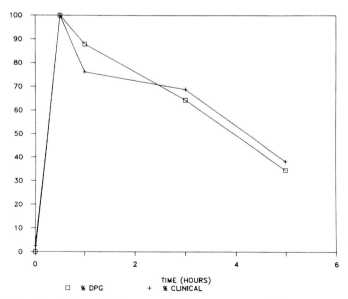

Figure 5. The relationship between DPG response and clinical response as percent of the one-half-hour reading. DPG response is the change in diastolic amplitude. The clinical response is prolongation of the time to exertion from stress testing.

As the blood vessels become more dilated, the energy of the bounce-back becomes greater in the finger. This is registered as an increase in diastolic amplitude.

Application to Nitroglycerin. Unpublished data have shown that doses of oral controlled-release nitroglycerin as low as 2.5 mg can produce a statistically significant change in DPG using only 12 subjects. DPG has been demonstrated to be linearly dose-dependent in five unpublished studies. This dose dependency has been independently corroborated by two other investigators.[3,9]

In a study using sublingual doses, DPG has been shown to correlate with nitroglycerin blood levels (r = 0.82, p <0.01). For buccal nitroglycerin, DPG profiles[7] are similar to clinical efficacy profiles.[10] Data from DPG and clinical studies have been plotted in Figure 5 as a percent change from the 30-minute readings to normalize the data in each study. The curves are strikingly similar over the five-hour test period. Because of this DPG/clinical relationship, DPG can be used to compare different formulations of nitroglycerin for relative effectiveness. It also means that DPG can potentially be used to compare the relative clinical effectiveness across different vasodilator drugs.

In summary, DPG is a relatively straightforward pharmacological response that is very sensitive to nitrate bioavailability. It is correlated to blood levels and clinical efficacy. This makes it an attractive candidate for conducting studies comparing vasodilators across formulations and across drugs.

PROLACTIN ELEVATION RESPONSE

Methodology. The phenothiazines are important drugs for treating mental and emotional illness. Not until recently have methods been available to determine blood levels of many of these drugs for single-dose bioavailability studies. Prior to the development of these assays, the rise in the prolactin level produced by phenothiazines was investigated as a tool for evaluating bioavailability.

The study of the mechanism of action of phenothiazine drugs indicates that they act through a blockade of dopaminergic receptors. This correlates with antipsychotic activity. Since dopaminergic neurons also tonically inhibit the release of prolactin from the pituitary gland, phenothiazines cause an increase in prolactin through dopaminergic blockade.[11] Thus, the rise in prolactin level not only can be used as an indication of drug bioavailability, but the rise can be used to evaluate clinical potency.

Application to Perphenazine. In a study designed to determine whether perphenazine produced a dose-dependent response, three subjects were treated with placebo, perphenazine 8 mg (one tablet), and perphenazine 16 mg (two 8 mg tablets) on three separate days. Prolactin blood levels were determined before dosing and at one, two, three, five, and eight hours. The mean results of the one- to eight-hour AUC of the prolactin response (Figure 6) were linear (r^2 = 0.996).[11] Although the small sample size warrants caution, statistical analysis reveals that a 20 percent difference between doses can be detected with 24 subjects (alpha = 0.05, beta = 0.20). This indicates the practicality of the response for bioavailability studies.

Additional studies on the prolactin response have been conducted on thioridazine and prochlorperazine (data on file, R.J. Erb, 1981). Preliminary results indicate dose-dependency for these drugs also.

SPECTRAL EDGE ANALYSIS OF ELECTROENCEPHALOGRAPHY

Methodology. In some cases, pharmacological data can be useful in determining relationships between blood levels and clinical response. One such study was designed to evaluate the relationship between blood levels for alprazolam and the EEG changes it produced.

EEG is a complex electrophysiological signal that offers numerous parameters for investigation. In this study, the spectral edge of the EEG was used as the pharmacological response. This parameter was used earlier by Hudson et al. to characterize the depth of anesthesia produced by thiopental. The spectral edge is defined as the frequency below which 95 percent of the EEG power is located. It provides an essentially continuous index of cerebral electrical activity and may be thought of as the highest frequency at which there is significant power.[12]

Application to Alprazolam. In this study, which illustrates the use of spectral edge, four subjects were each treated in a randomized four-way crossover study employing intravenous doses of placebo, alprazolam 0.5 mg bolus, alprazolam 2.0 mg bolus, and alprazolam 1.0 mg bolus followed by 72 μg/h infused over an eight-hour period for a total of 1.58 mg.

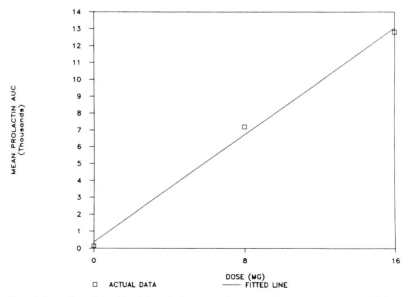

Figure 6. Dose-effect relationship of the prolactin response for perphenazine. Data are the mean AUC for three subjects for the rise in blood prolactin levels.

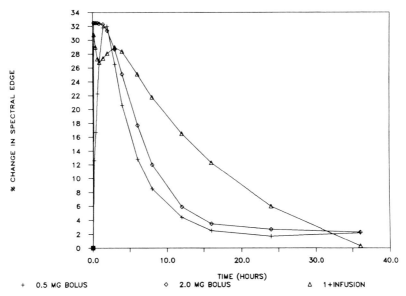

Figure 7. Placebo-corrected (P-C) spectral edge response for alprazolam and four subjects administered 0.5 mg, 2.0 mg, and 1.0 mg plus 72 μg/h for eight hours. Data were fitted by a smoothing five times.

The results of the spectral edge data are shown in Figure 7. Corresponding blood levels are shown in Figure 8. The blood level data indicated a dose-dependent response for the 0.5 and 2.0 mg doses. The constant infusion produced a plateau blood level during the eight-hour infusion. Comparing the spectral edge response with the blood level data revealed three things.

First, the 0.5 mg dose produced a peak response that is almost as high as the 2.0 mg response. This indicated that alprazolam effect on the spectral edge is on or near the plateau of maximum effect between the peak of 0.5 and 2.0 mg doses.

Second, examination of the AUC of the spectral edge response for the three doses indicated that the constant infusion provided the largest overall EEG response. This may provide additional clues for establishing dosing regimens.

Third, since the spectral edge response remained constant during the constant blood levels of the infusion, no tolerance to alprazolam was observed to develop for at least eight hours.

Thus, here is a case where a pharmacological study was used to provide clinically relevant information about a drug.

INFRARED THERMOGRAPHY

Methodology. The previous discussions of DPG, prolactin, and spectral edge are examples of pharmacological parameters developed to evaluate drugs that produce a specific type of pharmacological event.

The last pharmacological measurement to be discussed is infrared thermography, which measures a parameter that can be applied to a variety of drug product evaluations.

The thermographic method employs a video camera that is able to sense infrared radiation. Infrared rays are electromagnetic waves within the range of 0.7 to 1000 μ. This frequency is higher than radio waves and lower than visible light. Infrared rays are radiated spontaneously from any object that has a temperature above absolute zero. This radiation is related to the temperature of the object so that temperature of an object can be determined from the radiation it emits. Thus, a picture of the human body taken with an infrared camera is portraying a heat map of the surface of the body. Using computers, it is possible to quantitate selected areas of these pictures to within one-tenth of a degree centigrade.

Applications. The attribute of this methodology that makes it so useful for pharmaceutical research is that heat patterns are physical representations of underlying physiological processes. X-rays measure anatomical structure; infrared thermography depicts physiological events related to unseen pathological processes or drug activity. This makes the method potentially capable of generating data for a wide variety of pharmaceutical purposes including evaluation of:
- local or systemic vasodilators/vasoconstrictors;
- antiinflammatory activity;
- sunburn/sunscreen products;

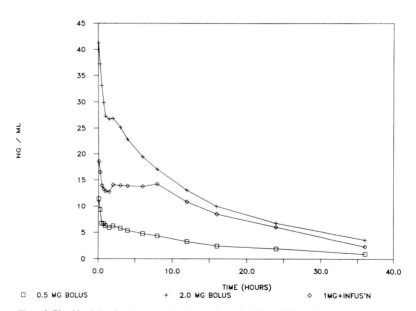

Figure 8. Blood level data for alprazolam for four subjects administered 0.5 mg, 2.0 mg, and 1.0 mg plus 72 μg/h for eight hours.

- potential sources of skin irritation;
- treatments for physical trauma;
- some pain-related processes.

In addition to having a variety of potential uses, thermography has the following positive attributes:

- it is a noncontact method;
- it causes no harmful complications;
- repeated measurements are quick and easy;
- it produces quantitative objective measurements.

The author has used thermography to evaluate beta-blocker activity, antiinflammatory activity, and the rate of delivery of a topically applied drug, and to establish a sports injury model for drug treatment efficacy evaluations.

Figure 9 is a sample illustration of the use of thermography for evaluating an antiarthritic drug. These data represent the change in temperature of an inflamed wrist during active drug and placebo treatments. During the first week, the active drug cooled the wrist by two degrees. During the placebo treatment, after a seven-day washout period, the wrist returned to its former state of inflammation.

Another example of the use of thermography is the determination of the vasodilatory effects of alpha-blockade by labetalol.[6] This hemodynamic response is primarily responsible for labetalol's blood pressure lowering effect and has the side benefit of eliminating the cold

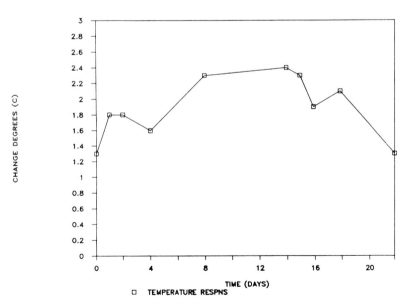

Figure 9. Antiinflammatory response in the wrist of one subject administered active (days 1–8) and placebo (days 14–22) drug for one week each. Treatments were separated by a seven-day washout period (days 8–14). The wrist cooled during active and warmed during placebo treatments. Parameter measured is the difference in temperature between the wrist and the forehead (control area).

extremities produced by other beta-blockers. Data collected over a four-hour period indicate that labetalol warms the hands as much as one full degree centigrade.

Summary

The use of pharmacological response data has been reviewed and examples have been sighted. In the general sense, some of the possible uses for quantifiable pharmacological responses discussed here include:
- determination of relative bioavailability;
- comparison of relative clinical potency;
- elucidation of clinical response kinetics;
- determination of drug tolerance;
- evaluation of clinical efficacy.

The use of pharmacological data will expand as technological advances allow more quantitative and reliable measurements of physiological processes to be made. As methods become more sophisticated, the now discernible boundaries between bioavailability, pharmacological response, and clinical efficacy will become much less distinct.

References

1. Code of federal regulations, title 21, food and drugs. Washington, DC: Office of the Federal Register, General Services Administration, April 1, 1977; paragraph 320.24, 117-8.
2. *Federal Register*, Aug. 26, 1977, vol. 42, no. 166, 43121-31.
3. IMHOF PR, OTT B, FRANKHAUSER P, CHU LC, HODLER J. Difference in nitroglycerin dose-response in venous and arterial beds. *Eur J Clin Pharmacol* 1980;*18*:445-60.
4. WINSOR T, KAYE H, MILLS B. Hemodynamic response of oral long-acting nitrates: evidence of gastrointestinal absorption. *Chest* 1972;*62*:407-13.
5. HANNEMANN RE, ERB RJ, STOLTMAN WP, et al. Digital plethysmography for assessing erythrityl tetranitrate bioavailability. *Clin Pharmacol Ther* 1981;*29*:35-9.
6. ERB RJ, PLACHETKA J. Thermographic evaluation of the peripheral vascular effects of labetalol and propranolol. *Cur Ther Res* 1985;*38*:68-73.
7. ERB RJ. Bioavailability of controlled release buccal and oral nitroglycerin by digital plethysmography. In: Stille G, Wagner W, Hermann W, eds. Advances in pharmacotherapy. vol. 1. Basel: Karger, 1982:35-43.
8. ERB RJ, STOLTMAN WP. Evaluation of two nitroglycerin dosage forms: a metered spray and a soft gelatin capsule. *J Pharmacokinet Biopharm* 1983;*11*:611-21.
9. PORCHET H, BIRCHER J. Digital plethysmography (DPG), a non-invasive method to assess the bioavailability of glyceryl trinitrate (abstract). *Experientia 1981;37*:674.
10. KAISER D, TEGEN W, LANGBEHN A, HOPPE M. Effect of buccal synchron nitroglycerin on pulmonary artery pressure at rest and during exercise. In: Stille G, Wagner W, Hermann W, eds. Advances in pharmacotherapy. vol. 1. Basel: Karger, 1982:73-97.
11. ERB RJ, STOLTMAN WP. Serum prolactin level increase in normal subjects following administration of perphenazine oral dosage forms: possible application to bioavailability testing. *J Pharm Sci* 1982;*71*:883-8.
12. HUDSON RJ, STANSKI DR, SAIDMAN LJ, MEATHE E. A model for studying depth of anesthesia and acute tolerance to thiopental. *Anesthesiology* 1983;*59*:301-8.

6. PHARMACOKINETIC / PHARMACODYNAMIC MODELING: STUDY DESIGN CONSIDERATIONS

Wayne A. Colburn

PHARMACOKINETIC/PHARMACODYNAMIC MODELING: STUDY DESIGN CONSIDERATIONS

Wayne A. Colburn

PHARMACOKINETICS AND PHARMACODYNAMICS are related. The only remaining question is. . .how? Based on the premise that an effect is a function of the amount and duration of free drug at a receptor or at the site of a biochemical event, it becomes clear that these direct or indirect effects can range from extremely simple to extremely complex temporal relationships between the pharmacokinetics in the sampled biofluid and the resulting pharmacodynamic effect. Historically the correlation of effects with blood concentrations has been poor for several reasons. Receptor sensitivities and disease state differences among patients, poorly defined clinical endpoints, the presence of active metabolites, and nonspecific and nonsensitive analytical methods explain some of the lack of direct correlation. However, there is also a myth that the time course of effects must parallel blood concentrations for a correlation to exist. Although the pharmacokinetic/pharmacodynamic relationships may be complex, they can be related using various pharmacokinetic/effector models together with certain effect equations. It is the purpose of this report to (1) elaborate these models and (2) to evaluate the various experimental study designs that can be used to identify and develop these pharmacokinetic/pharmacodynamic correlations to improve therapy.

Intrinsic Pharmacokinetics/Pharmacodynamics

For our purposes, the intrinsic pharmacokinetics of a drug are defined as the actual distribution, metabolism, and excretion characteristics associated with an instantaneous bolus dose. This is in contrast to those that are measured and, by definition, are subject to error. Beyond this, various drug input functions such as zero-order and first-order processes can be used to modify the intrinsic profile to achieve the input-modified pharmacokinetics of a drug. Similarly, the intrinsic pharmacodynamics are defined as the actual time course of effects, independent of any measurement error. It should be quite clear from these two definitions that the observed pharmacokinetic/pharmacodynamic profiles may be quite different from the intrinsic profiles, depending on the experimental design and the precision of pharmacokinetic and pharmacodynamic measures.

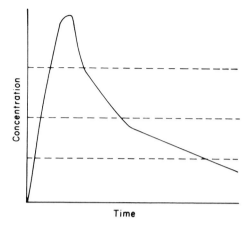

Figure 1. Representative plasma concentration-time profile used to show the importance of analytical sensitivity limits and sampling times on characterizing the pharmacokinetics of a drug and therefore developing pharmacokinetic/pharmacodynamic models.

Pharmacokinetic Models

ASSAY LIMITATIONS

Our ability to develop reasonable correlations of the pharmacokinetics and pharmacodynamics of any drug is no better than our least precise measure. In general, it is assumed that we are able to precisely measure the relevant plasma concentrations of a drug. However, this is not always the case. The recent literature contains several examples clearly indicating that multiple-dose predictions of certain drugs could not be accurately made from single-dose profiles due to analytical sensitivity limits.[1-4] If one cannot predict multiple-dose kinetic profiles from single-dose profiles, it is highly unlikely that pharmacokinetic/pharmacodynamic correlates can be determined.

Even with the most sensitive and specific analytical methods, it will not be possible to accurately correlate the biofluid and effect data unless the sampling schedule is appropriate to characterize the pharmacokinetic profile that elicits the effects. Figure 1 can be used to exemplify the points pertaining to both analytical sensitivity and sampling times.

In case 1, assume that the concentrations during the entire profile are capable of eliciting one or more quantifiable effects. However, if analytical sensitivity or biofluid sampling only allowed for detection of concentrations to the top line, then the ability to predict the effect could be limited if not totally prohibited, since effects would persist longer than plasma concentrations.

In case 2, assume that only the concentrations higher than the top hatched line are capable of eliciting the observed effect, and that assay sensitivity and/or sampling allowed measurements to the bottom hatched line. After a single dose, the ability to predict effect is supported by the pharmacokinetic data. However, on chronic dosing, the intuitive predictive ability would be lost as the lower, more sustained concentrations result in accumulation and a longer effective half-life of the drug.

STUDY DESIGN

Although both cases described above can be readily handled by the more complex modeling techniques to be discussed later, both would require appropriate study designs including adequate sampling times, improved analytical sensitivity, and/or additional multiple-dose regimens. This realization should only serve to clarify the need to develop adequate study designs if one is going to attempt to correlate observed effects with observed pharmacokinetic profiles.

APPROPRIATE MODEL

Once reliable analytical data and appropriate samples are available, the models we then use to fit the plasma or other biofluid data must reflect the absorption distribution metabolism excretion (ADME) of the drug of interest. If one is going to use the pharmacokinetic model to define the anticipated effects, the pharmacokinetic model must be able to describe the time course of the drug at the site(s) of action. This does not mean that the measured biofluid profile must parallel the effect profile, but rather that the measured biofluid profile can be used to predict the time course of effect. In the simplest case, the biofluid is the site of action. In more complex cases, the site of action may be in a tissue that is kinetically distinguished from the sampled biofluid. In this more complex situation, it is still possible to use the accurate biofluid profile, together with models to be discussed later, to predict the time course of effect.

INPUT FUNCTIONS

Drug input functions can dramatically influence the ability to measure and model the pharmacokinetic profile. As discussed previously, iv bolus dosing will result in the intrinsic pharmacokinetic profile which, together with adequate and appropriate assay and sampling methods, can yield a good approximation of this profile. However, alternate dosing methods such as zero-order iv infusion, first-order extravascular absorption from intramuscular, subcutaneous, or oral doses, or even first order iv infusions can influence this profile. Since these input functions affect the pharmacokinetic profile, they can be used under certain circumstances in single- and multiple-dose regimens to test the appropriateness of the pharmacokinetic/pharmacodynamic models. In addition, the first-order iv infusion input function will be discussed later for its rate-controlling characteristics and advantages it offers over both zero-order infusions and extravascular first-order input functions for model testing.

Thus, we can see from the above discussion that our ability to establish and develop a pharmacokinetic/pharmacodynamic correlation is highly dependent on our ability to accurately measure the relevant pharmacokinetic profile of the drug, and therefore is highly study-design dependent.

Pharmacodynamic Models

MODELING APPROACH

Two major approaches have been used to model the pharmacologic effects of drugs. The first approach establishes the percentages of patients that are subtherapeutic, therapeutic, and toxic across the observed concentration range of the drug of interest. This requires a large sample size from the total patient population. The second approach involves the correlation of graded responses with circulating drug or metabolite concentration in a smaller sample of the patient population of interest. Although both approaches provide valuable information for establishing and developing concentration-response relationships, this discussion will only deal with the latter modeling approach and will ultimately narrow the focus to combined pharmacokinetic/pharmacodynamic models.

DIRECT AND INDIRECT EFFECTS

Our ability to model the effect of a given drug is dependent on our ability to separate and ultimately to quantitate the beneficial and/or detrimental effects. Similarly, it is important that we are able to mechanistically separate direct and indirect effects. More importantly, it is imperative that we separate direct effects at peripheral sites of action from truly indirect biochemical mechanisms of action so that we can establish the correct concentration-effect relationships. Ultimately, then, the appropriate pharmacokinetic/pharmacodynamic models can be used to describe both single- and multiple-dose data as well as data from several routes of administration.

TYPES OF MODELS

Several concentration-effect equations have been used to describe the time course of pharmacologic effects of drugs. They include:
Linear model:

$$E = S \cdot C \qquad \text{(Eq. 1)}$$

where E = measured effect, S = linear coefficient, and C = drug concentration.

Sigmoid E_{max} model:

$$E = \frac{E_{max} \, C^s}{C_{ss}^{50^s} + C^s} \qquad \text{(Eq. 2)}$$

where E_{max} = maximum possible effect, C_{ss}^{50} = steady-state concentration at which effect is at half maximum, and s = power function. When s is equal to one, this model becomes the classical E_{max} model.

Baseline subtraction model:

$$E - E_o = \frac{E_{max} \, C}{C_{ss}^{50} + C} \qquad \text{(Eq. 3)}$$

where E_o = baseline effect. Equation 3 assumes that the baseline can be subtracted from the observed effect data leaving the 0–100 percent effect curve intact. However, in the case of the opioid analgesics and other compounds, endogenous substances bind to the receptor or interact biochemically to maintain the baseline effect. Under these circumstances, it is more likely that the baseline effects should be considered an integral part of the overall measured effect. The model will be referred to as the baseline inclusion model.

Baseline inclusion model:

$$E = \frac{E_{max}(C + Co)}{C_{ss}^{50} + (C + Co)} \tag{Eq. 4}$$

where Co = concentration of test substance that would be required to cause the baseline activity such that E includes the baseline effect. The conceptual basis of this approach is depicted in Figure 2 where the impact of baseline subtraction and baseline inclusion are shown schematically. Similarly, the influence of inadvertently using baseline subtraction when the baseline effect measures were the result of endogenous ligands is presented for two reasonable cases in Table 1. As one would expect, the influence of baseline subtraction was much greater at the lower end than at the upper end of the effect curve. This results in a significant difference in the observed C_{ss}^{50} as well as in the sigmoidicity parameter. It should be abundantly clear that application of the baseline subtraction method can result in erroneous parameter estimations and therefore erroneous pharmacokinetic/pharmacodynamic correlates. This equation form does not directly address the potential for endogenous baseline fluctuations during the course of the drug study; this aspect of the observed effects can be addressed using one or more placebo periods and allowing Co to vary during the time course of the study to accommodate the baseline fluctuations.

Alternate equation forms can be used that reflect indirect effects of a drug such as those involving biochemical events as follows:

$$E = Rsyn - Rdeg \tag{Eq. 5}$$

where the observed effect (E) reflects the rate of synthesis (Rsyn) and/or the rate of degradation (Rdeg) of some biochemically active substrate that can be influenced by the drug.

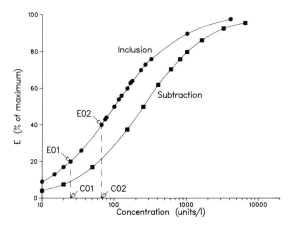

Figure 2. Schematic representation to show the importance of baseline inclusion and baseline subtraction on characterizing concentration-effect relationships.

Table 1. Influence of Baseline Inclusion and Baseline Subtracting on the Observed and Estimated Effect Parameters when the Baseline Effect is an Integral Part of the Observed Effect.

CASE 1			CASE 2		
CONCENTRATION	BI	BS	CONCENTRATION	BI	BS
0	20	0	0	40	0
10	26	8	10	44	7
50	43	29	33	50	17
100	56	45	100	63	38
125	60	50	167	70	50
150	64	55	200	73	55
300	76	70	400	82	71
1000	91	89	800	90	83
2000	95	94	1600	94	91
4000	98	97	3200	97	95

Case 1; Co $= 25$, $E_o = 20$, s $= 1$, $C_{ss}^{50} = 100$, $E_{max} = 100$
Case 2; Co $= 67$, $E_o = 40$, s $= 1$, $C_{ss}^{50} = 100$, $E_{max} = 100$
BI $=$ baseline inclusion; BS $=$ baseline subtracting.

Combined Models

Once the pharmacokinetics are well defined and appropriate pharmacologic endpoints have been elucidated, it is possible to combine them to create a pharmacokinetic/pharmacodynamic model in which an effector compartment is linked to the pharmacokinetic model (Figure 3). The effector compartment then drives the pharmacodynamic equation form. This approach has been previously described in detail and has been applied to a variety of compounds.[5,6] It has been possible to relate sampled biofluid concentrations to the observed effects of several compounds under a variety of dosing conditions. However, the ability to fit a set of data with a model does not mean that it is the correct model. Identifiability and uniqueness of the model require multiple inputs and/or both single- and multiple-dose predictability to validate the model for universal applicability; not just fitting one data set.

NONPARALLELISM

In many cases, once the appropriate effector equation has been combined with the pharmacokinetic/pharmacodynamic model, the observed effects still do not parallel the pharmacokinetic profile. The changes in observed effect lag behind the changes in drug concentration in the sampled site. This nonparallelism has been attributed to a partitioning lag between the sampled site and proposed site of action. Since inclusion of the effector compartment with the rate constant for elimination from effector site, K_{EO}, can account for this time shift, it is inferred that K_{EO} reflects the rate for partitioning to the effect site.[7]

Simulated data suggest, however, that even when the site of action is sampled, there can be a nonparallelism between drug concentration and effect. This observation has led this author to suggest alternatively that K_{EO} represents the rate constant for dissociation from the receptor rather than for partition from the sampled site to the site of action. The peripheral effect (Figure 3b) and specific tissue-effect models alluded to earlier[6] can readily separate tissue distribution from receptor occupancy.

PERIPHERAL EFFECT MODEL

The peripheral effect model (Figure 3b) allows one to explain data that otherwise cannot be adequately described. Apparent changes in pharmacokinetic/pharmacodynamic relationships as a function of route of administration or changing from single to multiple dosing can be explained on the basis of inappropriately fitting peripheral-effect data to a central-effect model.[6] It is imperative to choose the correct model in order to use the results to extrapolate to other modes and rates of administration.[8,9] In addition, choosing the appropriate peripheral effect model makes it possible to isolate factors that influence the time course of effect such as the kinetics of receptor binding, rather than to inappropriately attribute the time-dependent aspects to partitioning to the site of action.[6]

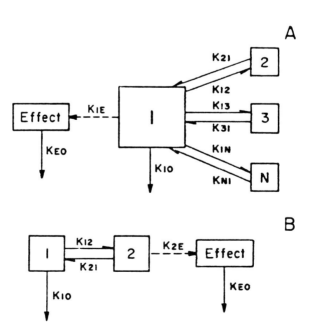

Figure 3. Pharmacokinetic/pharmacodynamic models for simultaneously fitting pharmacokinetics and pharmacologic effects. Scheme A is the conventional central effect model; B is the two-compartment peripheral effect model.

Experimental Design Considerations

As stated in the first section, both adequate and appropriate assay methods are required to define the intrinsic pharmacokinetics or drug input-modified pharmacokinetics of the drug of interest. In addition, it is critical to establish whether the effect mechanism is biochemical or receptor mediated to optimize sampling times for effect measurements. The pharmacologic end point(s) of interest must be readily quantifiable and relevant to therapy but need not be a direct measure of therapeutic effect. These measures can be either subjective or objective as long as they can be reproducibly quantified in the clinic. Finally, subject inclusion criteria must be sufficiently narrow to isolate the healthy subject or specific patient volunteer who is most appropriate to study the pharmacokinetic/pharmacodynamic correlates. For example, in cardiac failure, both acceptable and unacceptable concomitant medications must be considered and either conscientiously included or excluded in the protocol. An oversight of this type in the protocol design can result in unintelligible results from an otherwise perfectly designed study.

PATIENTS VS. NORMALS

One aspect of experimental design that must be considered from several perspectives is whether to use volunteer patients for whom the drug is intended or to use healthy volunteers. This topic has recently been reviewed[10] and only a brief overview follows: (1) what is the risk-to-benefit ratio for both study groups; (2) what will be the compliance of the two study groups under the intense sampling schedules required; and (3) can data from healthy volunteers be translated to the patient population of interest?

Once these questions have been answered, it should be self-evident which of the two study groups should be used for the drug of interest.

IMPROVING EFFECT MEASUREMENTS

In most cases, the variability of effect measures is greater than that of the pharmacokinetic measures. Therefore, extensive effect measures are required to minimize the influence of this variability on the modeling results. If one is convinced that the pharmacokinetic measures are more reliable than the pharmacodynamic measures, then sequential modeling (i.e., fitting pharmacokinetic data before the pharmacodynamic data) can be used to improve the overall modeling results. In addition, it has been shown that pooling effect measures can ultimately lead to the same conclusions.[11] Therefore, if the variability in the effect measures results in imprecise effect parameter estimates, pooling multiple-effect measures can help to resolve this problem.

Selection And Model Testing

The best time to develop the pharmacokinetic/pharmacodynamic modeling strategy is during early phase I tolerance studies in that this may be the only time that an investigator can approach the E_{max} value for certain drug effects. It is, therefore, the best time to test and understand the models. Although this may not always be possible, it should be our goal to attempt to begin pharmacokinetic/pharmacodynamic modeling as early as possible during the development of a drug. Early modeling, in the most ideal situation, involves testing the rates and routes of administration, various dose levels, and dosing regimens as well as investigating the influence of potentially active metabolites. Single-dose studies that control the rates and routes of administration as well as studies that control the transition from single to multiple doses can be used to establish and/or test the combined pharmacokinetic/pharmacodynamic models.

SINGLE-DOSE STUDIES

First-order and bolus iv dosing can be used in sequence to control and isolate the rate-limiting steps in the pharmacokinetic/pharmacodynamic model. The one-compartment open model can be used as an example. In this case, the following equations describe the plasma concentrations (C_p) and the hypothetical amount (A_E) in the effector compartment.

IV Bolus Dose.

$$C_p = \frac{X_o \, e^{-k_e t}}{V_p} \qquad \text{(Eq. 6)}$$

and

$$A_E = \frac{k_{1E} X_o}{(k_{EO} - k_e)} \, (e^{-k_e t} - e^{-k_{EO} t}) \qquad \text{(Eq. 7)}$$

Zero-Order IV Infusion.

$$C_p = \frac{k_o}{V_p k_e} \, (1 - e^{-k_e T}) \, e^{-k_e t'} \qquad \text{(Eq. 8)}$$

and

$$A_E = \frac{k_{1E} k_o}{k_e (k_{EO} - k_e)} \, (1 - e^{-k_e T}) \, e^{-k_e t'}$$
$$+ \frac{k_{1E} k_o}{k_{EO} (k_e - k_{EO})} \, (1 - e^{-k_{EO} T}) \, e^{-k_{EO} t'} \qquad \text{(Eq. 9)}$$

First-Order IV Infusion.

$$C_p = \frac{k_a \, X_o}{V_p \, (k_a - k_e)} \, (e^{-k_e t} - e^{-k_a t}) \qquad \text{(Eq. 10)}$$

and

$$A_E = \frac{k_{1E}k_aX_o}{(k_e - k_a)\,(k_{EO} - k_a)}\,e^{-k_a t} + \frac{k_{1E}k_aX_o}{(k_a - k_e)\,(k_{EO} - k_e)}\,e^{-k_e t}$$

$$+ \frac{k_{1E}k_a\,X_o}{(k_a - k_{EO})\,(k_e - k_{EO})}\,e^{-k_{EO} t} \qquad \text{(Eq. 11)}$$

where X_o = dose, V_p = volume of the plasma compartment, k_e = elimination rate constant, k_{1E} and k_{EO} = input and output rate constants for the effector compartment, k_o = zero-order input rate constant, k_a = first-order input rate constant, t = time, T = time during the zero-order infusion, and t ′ = time post zero-order infusion such that time t = T + t ′ during any zero-order infusion equations. There is no bioavailability term (F) since the complete dose is administered via the venous route. In this context, the ability to vary k_a and to guarantee that F = 1 is what makes this approach so useful.

Advantages of First-Order Input. Simple visual inspection of these equations shows the increased versatility of the first-order input form. For both the bolus and zero-order infusion forms, there is only one potentially rate-limiting term, k_e, for the pharmacokinetic portion of the model and only two potentially rate-limiting terms, k_e and k_{EO}, for the pharmacodynamic portion. In contrast, with the variable first-order infusion, there are two potentially rate-limiting terms, k_a and k_e, for the pharmacodynamic portion of the model and three potentially rate-limiting terms, k_a, k_{EO}, and k_e, for the pharmacodynamic. In addition, because k_a can be varied, it not only can be rate limiting, it can be rate controlling. In one limiting case, the iv bolus dose reflects k_a approaching infinity; whereas, in another case, k_a can be reduced so that it becomes slower than k_{EO} and/or k_e. It is readily apparent that by varying k_a, one can isolate rate limiting and/or controlling steps such that receptor kinetics can be separated from central/peripheral compartment pharmacokinetics. Although the one-compartment model was used in this case for the simplicity of the equation forms, it is obvious that greater application can be realized for the more complex multicompartment models. This conceptual approach to the problem has been previously described.[12] An example of this rate separation of effect for verapamil will be presented in the following section. The iv bolus can be used to establish the intrinsic pharmacokinetics of the compound and its resulting pharmacodynamics. The first-order iv infusion rate can then be sequentially controlled so that it ranges from the fastest to the slowest rate constant such that the dynamic parameters of the model can be isolated even if they would normally be hidden by the pharmacokinetic aspects of the model.

Finally, the effector equation for A_E is linked to the observed effect through the following E_{max} equation form:

$$E = \frac{[k_{EO}A_E/(k_{nE} \ V_n)] \ E_{max}}{(k_{EO}A_E/(k_{nE} \ V_n)] \ + \ C_{ss}^{50}} \qquad \text{(Eq. 12)}$$

where V_n = volume of the driving (nth) pharmacokinetic model compartment.

MULTIPLE-DOSE STUDIES

Once a model has been chosen based on single-dose data, it must be tested by accurately predicting the transition from single to multiple doses. It has been shown that even though an adequate fit of single-dose data can be obtained using several different models, if an inappropriate model has been chosen, the predicted and observed effects will systematically diverge as multiple doses are administered.[6] Although this procedure may not be universally applicable since some substances cause sensitivity or tolerance, relevant information should be obtainable even for these substances with short duration, low multiple-dose protocols.

Two types of routes of administration studies can be used to assess model selection.[13] The first evaluates the influence of rate and route on the concentration-effect profile.

Effect of Rate and Route of Administration. An example of this type of study exists for verapamil where the investigators were unable to explain the discrepancy in the concentration-effect relationship as

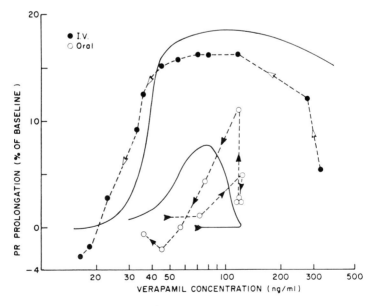

Figure 4. Verapamil plasma concentrations and observed effects reported by Reiter et al.[12] as well as simulated plasma concentration and effects using a two-compartment central effect model (adapted from Reference 13).

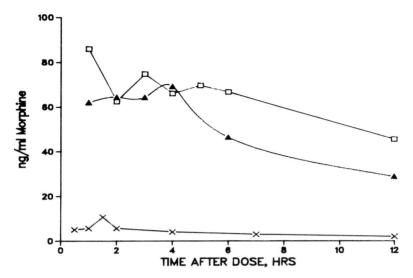

Figure 5. Time course of plasma concentrations and cerebrospinal fluid (CSF) concentrations following systemic im administration (plasma and CSF) and local peridural application (plasma and CSF) of morphine (modified and adapted from Reference 16).

a function of iv bolus, iv infusion, and oral dosing.[14] Subsequently, we have been able to provide a possible explanation for the influence of route of administration on concentration-effect relationships (Figure 4) [12,13] using a pharmacokinetic/pharmacodynamic model.[15] Other investigators have postulated that these differences are due to non-specific assay methods[16] and/or stereospecific first-pass metabolism.[17] However, the first-order iv infusion method described earlier can be used to isolate the true mechanism by which these apparent route-dependent effects occur. If stereospecific metabolism and nonspecific assays account for the different pharmacokinetic/pharmacodynamic relationships, then an iv bolus and a first-order iv infusion will result in identical concentration-effect relationships for both modes of administration. However, if the rate-limiting first-order input is the cause of the different pharmacokinetic/pharmacodynamic relationships, then these two iv modes of administration will result in different concentration-effect relationships in spite of the identical route of administration. Although the mechanism responsible for this discrepancy may not be this simple (e.g., it may involve both rate and route), this approach should help to answer the question.

Local Administration. The second type of study evaluates the pharmacokinetic/pharmacodynamic model as a function of local administration. These studies can be particularly useful in delineating appropriate models for narcotic/opioid analgesics as well as other substances that can be administered for localized effects. The drug of interest can be administered locally by the epidural, peridural, subarachnoid, as well as other routes and the effects can be compared to the effects observed following systemic (oral, intramuscular, subcutaneous, or iv) doses. Using this approach, it should be possible to isolate a peripheral effect compartment such as the central nervous system (CNS) and to more precisely determine the distribution characteristics as well as specific effect parameters such as the association and dissociation rate constants. An example of this type of local effect is shown in Figure 5.[16] Morphine readily distributes into the CNS, and therefore the CNS can be considered part of the routinely sampled plasma compartment. However, following local administration by the epidural route, morphine concentrations in the CNS are much higher at equivalent plasma concentrations than they are following systemic (intramuscular) administration.[18] This observation can be used to advantage therapeutically, and must be considered and used to advantage when developing pharmacokinetic/pharmacodynamic models for these types of compounds.

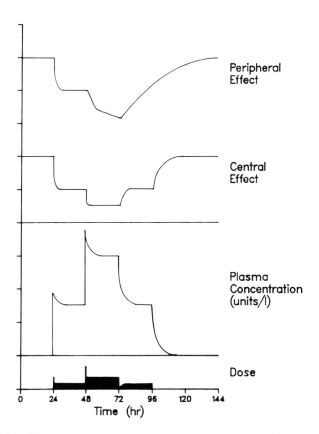

Figure 6. A graphic representation to show the influence of direct central and peripheral receptor effects during a cascade input function. For the central receptor, the same steady-state drug concentration elicits the same effect; for the peripheral receptor it does not.

Cascade Dosing Regimen. A cascade dosing regimen can be used to evaluate the concentration-effect relationship. This type of dose/concentration profile is shown schematically in Figure 6. A placebo period is used to establish the baseline effect followed by two escalating bolus infusion doses followed by a return to the initial dose and finally back to placebo. The concentrations and steady states associated with each dose level are used to confirm dose proportionality and time-independence of the pharmacokinetic profile. Two effect profiles are shown: case 1 represents the situation where the cascade confirms a central effect in that equivalent steady-state concentrations elicit the same effect. Case 2 represents a situation where the cascade confirms a noncentral effect where the same steady-state concentrations elicit distinctly different effect profiles. The example shown here reflects iv dosing, but this approach can also be used for oral dosing using a loading- and maintenance-dose approach to achieve the goal.

TOLERANCE MODELS

Narcotic analgesics, benzodiazepines, and certain other drugs cause tolerance to develop during chronic dosing. For these compounds, it is possible to employ the same cascade approach but over a significantly shorter period of time. This requires elaborate loading-dose schemes to achieve and adjust steady states within a few hours. In addition to this approach, one should develop a tolerance model for these types of compounds that could subsequently be used to adjust doses and rotate the drugs administered so that optimum therapy could be maintained. These models would incorporate time-dependent functions to modify the effect parameters k_{1E}, k_{EO}, C_{ss}^{50}, o, and/or E_{max}. Levy and coworkers have used this approach to model enzyme induction pharmacokinetics, which is similar to the development of tolerance in effect modeling.[19,20] Although it has been stated previously,[5,6] k_{1E} is not important to the effect modeling because it mathematically cancels out of the calculations in this model. It is included here because an alternate model will be developed in the subsequent section where both k_{1E} and k_{EO} are important in the effector equation. In either event, time-dependent changes in the pharmacokinetic or the pharmacodynamic parameters can be incorporated into the equation(s) to accommodate pharmacokinetic and/or pharmacodynamic changes that occur during repeated dosing. The basis for the similarity in approaches is that both enzyme and receptor changes occur as a result of change in protein synthesis and therefore the time course reflects protein elimination.[19,20]

ACTIVE METABOLITES

Metabolites formed from the administered compound can also elicit desired or undesired effects. These metabolites can behave as agonists or antagonists; they can compete for the same receptor and/or can occupy other receptors. To model these effects one must be able to administer and measure the metabolite(s) as well as the parent compound. Once this has been done, the principle of additive receptor occupancy can be used to quantitate the observed effects and then to predict the anticipated effects. It cannot be assumed that drug and metabolite have the same receptor binding characteristics and it must not be assumed that observed effects are additive. The temporal aspects of these interactions must be considered when both a drug and its metabolite(s) are involved in the observed effect. A metabolite that differs from parent drug with respect to rates on and off the receptor, distribution characteristics, and elimination profile (i.e., slower) will impart different observed effects early in the time course in the presence of the parent drug than it will later when the parent drug has been almost totally eliminated. However, this can be readily accommodated by the combined parent/metabolite modeling approach described herein.

Prediction of Dosing Regimen

Once the appropriate pharmacokinetic/pharmacodynamic model and effector equations have been resolved, various dosing regimens can be evaluated to determine the most appropriate doses and dosing intervals to achieve a desired endpoint: maximization of desired effects while minimizing undesirable effects. Meffin and coworkers have used this approach with the antiarrhythmic drug tocainide.[21] If one were able to establish the concentration-effect relationship for both the desired and undesired effects of a drug, it would be possible to predict the therapeutic windows for a variety of regimens such as those shown in Figure 7. This figure illustrates observed effects of steady-state plasma concentrations following 1200 mg qd, 600 mg bid, and 300 mg qid dosing of a hypothetical one-compartment drug with a 12-hour elimination half-life. The relationship between dosing interval and effect is

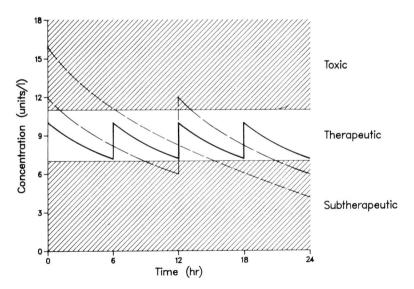

Figure 7. Schematic representation and observed effects of steady-state plasma concentrations following 1200 mg qd, (----) 600 mg bid (— —), and 300 mg qid (——) dosing of a hypothetical one-compartment drug with a 12-hour elimination half-life.

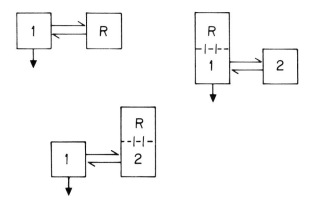

Figure 8. A schematic representation of three receptor models where the receptor kinetics can influence the pharmacokinetics depending on the amount and the on and off rate constants for the receptors. The models represent cases where the receptor causes the biexponential profile or where the receptor becomes the third exponential in the pharmacokinetic profile.

obvious for the same total daily dose. A 600 mg po bid dosing regimen for this same drug with an absorption half-life of two to three hours would maintain therapeutic concentrations throughout the day. A 1200 mg po controlled-release dosage form with an absorption half-life of six hours could be administered once daily to achieve the same goal.

After predicting a series of optimal regimens, only the most promising could be tested in a patient population to minimize exposure to drug as well as to minimize adverse effects while optimizing efficacy. As was the case for the single-dose situation, the investigator should make an effort to cover the entire effect curve from EO to E_{max} during evaluation of multiple-dose regimens.

Alternative Models

The models described herein reflect the approach first described by Sheiner et al.[5] This modeling approach revolves around the concept that the distribution of the drug to the effector compartment is non-destructive; i.e., drug entering or leaving the effector compartment does not influence the pharmacokinetic profile of the drug. A more realistic approach to this problem is to assume that drug binding to the receptor does influence the pharmacokinetic profile, albeit only to a negligible extent, and therefore that both k_{1E} and k_{EO} are integral parts of the effector compartment time-course. An example of this approach where a one-compartment pharmacokinetic model has a single effector compartment has been reported earlier[12] and is shown in Figure 8. It should be clear from this model that the equations that describe the effector/receptor compartment are identical to those of the peripheral compartment for a two-compartment model. The only difference here is that the effector/receptor on and off rates are generally fast compared to the pharmacokinetic rate constants and the volume of the effector/receptor compartment is generally extremely small compared to the pharmacokinetic compartment. This can be described as follows:

$$C_p = \frac{X_o\,(k_{EO} - \alpha)}{V_p\,(\beta - \alpha)} \quad e^{-\alpha t} + \frac{X_o\,(k_{EO} - \beta)}{V_p\,(\alpha - \beta)} \quad e^{-\beta t} \quad \text{(Eq. 13)}$$

$$A_E = \frac{k_{1E}\,X_o}{(\beta - \alpha)} \quad (e^{-\beta t} - e^{-\alpha t}) \quad \text{(Eq. 14)}$$

Again, the difference between this model and that previously described is the implicit involvement of both k_{1E} and k_{EO} in the effector compartment time course. In addition, although a simple case was used as an example, this approach can be applied to the central compartment effects of more complex pharmacokinetic models or even to peripheral compartment effects of multicompartment models using caternary modeling techniques. The first-order iv dosing techniques described earlier should be very useful in isolating both the pharmacokinetic and the pharmacodynamic parameters for this type of model.

PEAK EFFECT PRECEDES PEAK CONCENTRATION

In general, the time course of the effect has been concomitant with or delayed in relation to the plasma concentration, and current models are based on correlating these effects with sampled venous blood concentrations. The concurrent or time-delayed temporal nature of these effects made the venous equilibrium model conceptually pleasing. However, as one peruses the literature, it becomes apparent that in certain cases the effect-time profiles precede those of the plasma concentra-

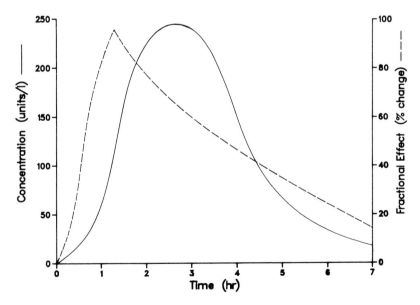

Figure 9. A concentration (—)/effect (---) profile wherein the effect precedes the plasma drug concentration profile. This type of profile can reflect venous sampling when, in fact, the arterial concentration drives the effect component.

tions.[22,23] A schematic representation of this type of phenomenon is presented in Figure 9, which shows that the maximum effect occurs before the maximum plasma concentration.

One begins to question whether there is an active first-pass metabolite or another process that could cause this anomaly. Certainly an active first-pass metabolite that precedes the measured drug into the systemic circulation and site of action could cause this phenomenon. However, in the absence of an active metabolite, venous as opposed to arterial sampling could cause the same unanticipated effect profile. Current venous sampling models can accommodate these observations if a time-delay function is incorporated into these models. However, the exact relationship between plasma concentration and effect as well as the predictive capability from one mode of administration to another can only be accomplished using arterial blood sampling and modeling.

Summary

Pharmacokinetic/pharmacodynamic modeling must: (1) reduce the pharmacokinetic and pharmacodynamic observations to a readily communicable form, and (2) predict future events by other modes of administration. Several approaches have been reviewed with an emphasis on the hypothetical-effect compartment models. Methods of developing and evaluating the model, including comparison of observed effects as a function of rate and route of administration as well as both single and multiple doses, were presented. It was shown that good estimates of intrinsic or input-controlled pharmacokinetic profile as well as the intrinsic pharmacodynamic profile are necessary to make good use of pharmacokinetic/pharmacodynamic modeling techniques, and that these goals are achievable only with adequate experimental study designs.

References

1. SIDDOWAY LA, MCALLISTER CB, WILKINSON GR. Amiodarone dosing: a proposal based on its pharmacokinetics. *Am J Heart* 1983;*106*:951-6.

2. RIVA E, AARONS L, LATINI R. Amiodarone kinetics after single iv bolus and multiple dosing in healthy volunteers. *Eur J Clin Pharmacol* 1984;*27*:491-4.

3. MASSARELLA J, VANE F, BUGGE C, et al. Etretinate kinetics during chronic dosing in severe psoriasis. *Clin Pharmacol Ther* 1985;*37*:439-46.

4. COLBURN WA, INTURRISI CE. D-propoxyphene: accumulation or altered kinetics. *Eur J Clin Pharmacol* 1985;*28*:725-6.

5. SHEINER LB, STANSKI DR, VOZEH S, et al. Simultaneous modeling of pharmacokinetics and pharmacodynamics: application to d-tubocurarine. *Clin Pharmacol Ther* 1979;*25*:358-71.

6. COLBURN WA. Simultaneous pharmacokinetic and pharmacodynamic modeling. *J Pharmacokinet Biopharm* 1981;*9*:367-88.

7. HOLFORD NHG, SHEINER LB. Kinetics of pharmacologic response. *Pharmacol Ther* 1982;*16*:143-66.

8. GONDA I, MARPUR ES. Accumulation in the peripheral compartment of a linear two-compartment open model. *J Pharmacokinet Biopharm* 1980;*8*:99-104.

9. WEISS M. On pharmacokinetics in target tissue. *Biopharm Drug Dispos* 1985;*6*:57-66.

10. BRAZZELL RK, COLBURN WA. Choosing populations for pharmacokinetic studies. *J Clin Pharmacol* 1986;*26*:242-7.

11. HOLAZO AA, BRAZZELL RK, COLBURN WA. Pharmacokinetic and pharmacodynamic modeling of cibenzoline plasma concentrations and antiarrhythmic effect. *J Clin Pharmacol* 1986;*26*:336-45.

12. COLBURN WA. Do pharmacokinetics or receptor kinetics determine the pharmacodynamics of the benzodiazepines? (abstract). *J Pharm Sci* 1984:*73*:P8.

13. GODFREY KR, JONES RP, BROWN RF. Identifiable pharmacokinetic models: the role of extra inputs and measures. *J Pharmacokinet Biopharm* 1980;*8*:633-48.

14. REITER MJ, SHAND DG, PRITCHETT ELC. Comparison of intravenous and oral verapamil dosing. *Clin Pharmacol Ther* 1982;*32*:711-20.

15. COLBURN WA, BRAZZELL RK, HOLAZO AA. Verapamil pharmacodynamics following iv and oral doses: theoretical considerations. *J Clin Pharmacol* 1986;*26*:71-3.

16. EICHELBAUM M, MIKUS G, VOGELGESANG B. Pharmacokinetics of $(+)-$, $(-)-$, and $(+/-)-$ verapamil after intravenous administration. *Br J Clin Pharmacol* 1984;*17*:453-8.

17. VOGELGESANG B, ECHIZEN H, SCHMIDT E, et al. Stereoselective first-pass metabolism of highly cleared drugs: studies of the bioavailability of L-and D-verapamil examined with a stable isotope technique. *Br J Clin Pharmacol* 1984;*18*:733-40.

18. BELLANCA L, LATTERI MT, LATTERI S, et al. Plasma and CSF morphine concentrations after im and epidural administration. *Pharmacol Res Commun* 1985;*17*:189-96.

19. LEVY RH, LAI AA, DUMAIN MS. Time-dependent kinetics. IV. Pharmacokinetic theory of enzyme induction. *J Pharm Sci* 1979;*68*:398-9.

20. LEVY RH, DUMAIN MS, COOK JL. Time-dependent kinetics. V. Time course of drug levels during enzyme induction (one-compartment model). *J Pharmacokinet Biopharm* 1979;*7*:557-78.

21. MEFFIN PJ, WINKLE RA, BLASCHKE TF, et al. Response optimization of drug dosage: antiarrhythmic studies with tocainide. *Clin Pharmacol Ther* 1977;*22*:42-57.

22. JAVAID JI, FUCHIMAN MW, SCHUSTER CR, et al. Cocaine plasma concentrations: relation to physiological and subjective effects in humans. *Science* 1978;*202*:227-8.

23. ALOUSI AA, IWAN T, EDELSON J, et al. Correlation of hemodynamic and pharmacokinetic profile of milrinone in the anesthetized dog. *Arch Int Pharmacodyn* 1984;*267*:59-66.

7. POPULATION PHARMACOKINETICS: APPLICATION TO CLINICAL TRIALS

Thaddeus H. Grasela, Jr.

POPULATION PHARMACOKINETICS:
APPLICATION TO CLINICAL TRIALS

Thaddeus H. Grasela, Jr.

IN THE EARLIEST PHARMACOKINETIC STUDIES, the primary objective was the estimation of the parameters of a pharmacokinetic model that had been developed to describe the concentration-time course of a drug in plasma or urine. The object of study was the individual, and pharmacokinetic studies were designed to yield the maximum amount of information regarding the pharmacokinetic disposition of a drug in the individual.

As the field developed, pharmacokinetic techniques began to be used to explore the relationships between physiology and drug disposition. Pharmacokinetic studies were performed in order to determine how drug disposition was affected by various disease states, by patient characteristics such as age and weight, and by interacting drugs. This has resulted, in many cases, in improved patient care and a reduction in iatrogenically-induced drug toxicity.

This change in emphasis in pharmacokinetics has also been accompanied by a change in the focus of these studies. Estimating individual pharmacokinetic parameters has given way to determining the typical pharmacokinetic behavior of a drug in a population of patients. Until recently, however, the same techniques used to perform individual pharmacokinetic studies have simply been adapted for use in determining population paramters. There are a number of disadvantages to this approach, however, that limit the usefulness of the information obtained, and these will be discussed.

In recent years, an alternative approach to estimating population pharmacokinetic parameters has been developed. This approach, implemented in the computer program, NONMEM, has been advocated by Sheiner et al. as an alternative to traditional pharmacokinetic studies when the population, as opposed to the individual, is the object of study.[1]

The objectives of this paper are to: (1) briefly compare and contrast the traditional vs. the NONMEM approach to estimating population pharmacokinetic parameters; (2) review the results of analyses of simulated and clinical data that explore the performance of NONMEM in analyzing nonexperimental data; and (3) discuss the incorporation of the NONMEM approach into clinical trials and offer suggestions for the effective utilization of NONMEM in this setting.

Population Pharmacokinetic Parameters

There are three basic types of population pharmacokinetic parameters. Fixed-effect parameters quantify the population average kinetics of a drug (e.g., the population mean clearance or volume of distribution, V_d), and the relationships between pharmacokinetics and physiology (e.g., the relationship between drug clearance and creatinine clearance). The second type of population parameter, the interindividual random-effect parameter, quantifies the typical magnitude of interindividual variability in pharmacokinetic parameters. The third type of population parameter, the intraindividual random-effect parameter, quantifies the typical magnitude of the intraindividual (residual error) variability.[1]

UTILITY OF POPULATION PHARMACOKINETIC PARAMETERS

Pharmacokineticists are comfortable with thinking of clearance and volume of distribution as population parameters. However, when describing the population characteristics of a drug, the variability of clearance and the magnitude of intraindividual variability must also be thought of as distinct population parameters. Accurate estimates of these parameters, fixed and random, are important for a number of clinically relevant reasons.

Dosing Guidelines. The population mean clearance and volume of distribution are useful in developing dosing guidelines for patients who receive the drug for therapeutic indications. The interindividual variability of these parameters provides a means of assessing the degree of confidence an investigator or clinician can have when recommending dosing guidelines from mean clearance and volume of distribution data. The variability parameters can also be used to determine the urgency and frequency of follow-up of the patient. Moreover, interpretation of measured drug levels in patients and subsequent dosage adjustment, using, for example, Bayesian forecasting techniques, requires knowledge of both fixed- and random-effect parameters.[2]

Bioavailability Assessment. The population characteristics of bioavailability are of particular interest to drug companies and drug regulatory agencies. Mean bioavailability of a preparation is obviously important. Of equal importance, however, is the variability in bioavailability. If the variability in the extent of absorption is very great, even if the mean bioavailability of the preparation is 100 percent, the product may not be acceptable for use in patients.

Setting Direction For Further Study. Population pharmacokinetic parameters can also serve as a guide for future drug studies. For example, a large degree of unexplained interindividual variability in an otherwise homogeneous population may suggest that other factors, as yet undetermined, may be affecting the pharmacokinetics of the drug.

Traditional Approaches

NAIVE POOLED DATA METHOD

In the past, two methods have traditionally been used to determine population pharmacokinetic parameters. One approach, the naive pooled data (NPD) method, pools plasma concentration-time data from many individuals, creating in effect a single (mega) individual. This approach ignores the differences in kinetics between individuals, which is in itself an immediate disadvantage. Furthermore, this approach has been consistently shown to yield inaccurate and imprecise estimates of population pharmacokinetic parameters.[3,4] Thus, this approach should generally not be used and it will not be considered further in this discussion.

STANDARD TWO-STAGE METHOD

A second, more commonly employed approach, has been referred to as the standard two-stage (STS) method. As the name implies, determination of population parameters proceeds in two stages. In the first stage, an appropriate study protocol is implemented to allow determination of pharmacokinetic parameters for individual subjects. This typically involves administering an intravenous dose of drug followed by intensive plasma and/or urine sampling. The resulting concentration-time profile is then analyzed using nonlinear regression techniques to provide pharmacokinetic parameter estimates for the individual subjects. In the second stage, these individual estimates are pooled to provide the population pharmacokinetic parameter estimates.[5]

Although there are a number of important advantages to this approach, the clinical utility of these parameters may be seriously limited because of the source of the data. The subjects are very often normal volunteers or patients with mild degrees of illness who have been recruited for the study. Major problems can arise when one attempts to extrapolate results obtained from these volunteers to patients receiving the drug for therapeutic effect.

The difficulty lies in the sampling requirements of traditional pharmacokinetic studies. Serious ethical questions arise when one attempts to perform these studies in critically ill, pediatric, and elderly patients who may not be able to tolerate the rigors of a traditional pharmacokinetic study. Other problems with this approach include the small number of subjects studied, the cost of these studies, and the fact that the rigid experimental protocol will prevent the discovery of factors such as diet or drug-drug interactions that may have a clinically significant effect on pharmacokinetics.

The problem, then, is how one can obtain reasonable (i.e., accurate and precise) estimates of population pharmacokinetic parameters in these patient populations of interest.

NONMEM Approach

An approach to this problem, which has been advocated by Sheiner et al., involves the use of fragmentary data generated as part of the routine clinical care of the patient or collected during phase III clinical trials. They have proposed that this data, consisting of the patient's drug dosing history (i.e., time of drug administration, route, dose, and formulation) in conjunction with randomly obtained drug concentrations and, perhaps, supplemented with additional samples obtained without affecting patient care, can provide valuable information regarding drug disposition.[1]

ADVANTAGES

Sheiner and Beal have described several advantages to the use of this data. First, the data are representative since they are gathered from those individuals comprising the population of interest. Second, the ethical problems of performing research on critically-ill patients are nonexistent since the data are already being generated as part of patient care. Third, the data are inexpensive since most costs are absorbed in the justifiable expense of patient care or the performance of the phase III trial. Finally, serendipity is possible.[5] A variety of concomitant drugs, diets, and so forth will be represented in the data base, and, with careful analysis, clues to the effects of such factors should be uncovered.

PROBLEMS IN DATA ANALYSIS

Reliability of Data. In the past, data analysts have been reluctant to handle such data, and with good reason. As Sheiner and Beal pointed out, there are a number of serious problems that arise when one attempts to analyze routine clinical data. The reliability of the data is now suspect since patient compliance, timing of doses, and plasma sampling may not be known very accurately. A number of different laboratories, using different methodologies, may be performing the assays. The patient population will be very heterogeneous, and some patients may be very unstable and have rapidly shifting kinetic parameters. In addition, since there is effectively no study design, plasma samples will not be obtained at the most efficient times to allow accurate parameter estimation.[5]

Error Structure. In addition to the problems with the quality of data, there are also serious problems in data analysis. When ordinary least squares is used to obtain estimates of the individual's pharmacokinetic parameters, it is implicitly assumed that all errors intervening between the "true" level and the observed level are: (1) independent, (2) additive, and (3) of the same typical magnitude. As discussed by Sheiner and Beal, all of these assumptions are open to question even when analyzing experimental data.[5] Measurement (assay) error, for example, often begins at a lower limit of detectability and then rises, often in proportion to the drug concentration. In an effort to adjust for the increase in error magnitude associated with higher true values, data analysts often resort to weighting the data by the reciprocal of the concentration or of the concentration squared. Because of the quality and quantity of data available from traditional pharmacokinetic studies, this approach provides a reasonable balance. When analyzing routine clinical data, however, no easy adjustment for the variable error magnitude is available.

Estimation Error. Figure 1 illustrates the problem that can occur when inadequate and misleading data are used to estimate pharmacokinetic parameters.[6] In Figure 1a, the dashed line represents a least squares fit to some data collected over a reasonable period of time. In this case, the fitted line is reasonably close to the true (solid) line. In Figure 1b, however, the line obtained using a particularly poor sampling of the data results in a markedly different fit. Since the data points sampled might be just as likely to have yielded a steeper slope, the population mean fit to the data might not be biased. However, the estimates of the population interindividual variability of the parameters will be biased upwards. These estimates will be contaminated with both real interindividual variability and the variability in estimating the parameters. The consequences of this problem are illustrated by the results of the simulation discussed below.

In light of these problems, it is clear that a more complex data analysis approach will be required than the standard one. An approach that can be used is the method of extended least squares as applied to a non-linear mixed-effect statistical model.[1] The application of this approach to pharmacokinetic parameter estimation is actually an approximate maximum likelihood method. This approach was originally developed by scientists and statisticians in econometrics and sociology, who are also faced with the same problems: the analysis of nonexperimental "naturalistic" data.[7] A description of the extended least-squares approach and its relationship to ordinary or weighted least squares is available in Reference 5.

DISADVANTAGES

Model Specification. Although the ability to extract population pharmacokinetic parameters from clinical data represents a significant advantage, there are some disadvantages associated with this approach.

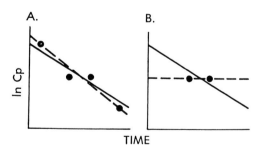

Figure 1. Effect of estimation error on population pharmacokinetic parameters. A monoexponential rate constant is to be fit to drug concentration (Cp) vs. time data. This constant is the negative slope of the linear function of log Cp vs. time. In both panels, some (Cp,t) data for an individual is plotted as points; the "true" function for the individual is plotted as the solid line, while the fitted line, using ordinary least squares (OLS), is plotted as the dashed line.

a. Four (Cp,t) values spanning a reasonable time range are available. Despite small deviations of observation from true values (due to measurement error), the OLS fit is close to the true value.

b. Only the least informative two of the four points in panel A are available: Now the OLS fit is very wrong because it regards the available points as though they were true values (reprinted with permission from Reference 6).

The complex nature of the data requires that one write explicit statistical error models, which must then be incorporated into the pharmacokinetic model. These pharmacostatistical models can be quite complicated; and if sufficient care is not exercised, unfortunate errors can result that are not easily detected. The process of specifying these statistical models has been described elsewhere and will not be discussed here.[1]

Limited Experience. The second, although certainly only temporary, disadvantage of NONMEM is the lack of experience with this program in biomedical situations. Until recently, there was very little information in the literature regarding the application of NONMEM to clinical problems, and it was unclear how population pharmacokinetic studies should be designed. In the last several years, however, studies have begun to appear in which NONMEM was used to perform a population analysis. These studies have examined the population pharmacokinetic characteristics of digoxin,[1] procainamide,[8] phenytoin,[9] phenobarbital,[10] and warfarin.[11]

Comparative Analysis of Simulated Data

MICHAELIS-MENTEN AND BIEXPONENTIAL MODELS

Recently, Sheiner and Beal have performed several simulation studies comparing the performance of NONMEM with the two traditional methods for estimating population parameters, the NPD method and the STS method. The first simulation compared the ability of the methods to estimate the parameters of a Michaelis-Menten type model from routine clinical pharmacokinetic data concerning phenytoin.[3] The second simulation compared the ability of the methods to estimate parameters of a biexponential model from experimental pharmacokinetic data.[4]

The results of these investigations yielded similar conclusions. The NPD method was distinctly inferior to the two other methods in all respects. The STS method was either comparable to or sometimes inferior to the NONMEM method with respect to estimating fixed-effect parameters and intraindividual random-effect parameters. The NONMEM method was markedly superior to the STS method for estimating interindividual random-effect parameters.

MONOEXPONENTIAL MODEL

A third study compared the performance of NONMEM and the STS method in estimating the parameters of a simple monoexponential kinetic model from routine clinical pharmacokinetic data. Although not specifically designed to answer questions regarding study design, this simulation provides some useful information that can be used in planning a population study involving the collection of routine clinical data.

Methods. The following description of the method used to perform the simulation is abstracted from Reference 12. The data were assumed to arise from regular repetitive (bolus) dosing to a monoexponential structural model:

$$Cp_{ij*} = \frac{De^{(-k_jt_{ij})} (1-e^{(-n_{ij}k_jt_{ij})})}{V_{dj} (1-e^{-k_j\tau})} \qquad \text{Eq. 1}$$

where Cp_{ij*} = true drug concentration in the jth individual, D = dose given to each individual; V_{dj} = volume of distribution of the drug for the jth individual; $k_j = Cl_j/V_{dj}$, where Cl_j = clearance of the drug in the jth individual; t_{ij} = time associated with the Cp_{ij*}, measured as time since the last previous dose; n_{ij} = interdose interval associated with Cp_{ij*} (the nth interdose interval occurs between doses n and n + 1); and τ = length of the interdose interval.

Individual values for clearance were randomly selected from a log-normal distribution of clearance values having a mean of 0.693 and a coefficient of variation of 50 percent. The individual's V_d was randomly chosen from a log-normal distribution of V_d values with a mean of 1.0 and a coefficient of variation of 30 percent.

For all simulations, $\tau = 1$ and dose = 1 so that the units of time are drug half-lives. By choosing appropriate values for t_{ij} and n_{ij} (see below), the individual parameters were used to compute Cp_{ij*}. Intra-individual error was then randomly selected from a log-normal distribution with a mean of zero and a coefficient of variation of 15 percent and added to the true value. These simulated measured values were then analyzed using the STS method and NONMEM and the results were compared.

In addition to comparing these methods, the influence of certain "design" factors in the routine data, such as the tradeoff between increasing the number of individuals vs. increasing the number of samples from each individual, were examined. This was accomplished by specifying various design parameters, i.e., the interdose interval (n_j), the sampling times after a dose (t_{ij}), the number of samples per subject (m_j), and the number of individuals (n). In the basic design used to generate a baseline data set for comparing methods and alternative data designs, the Cp for each individual was chosen to represent samples drawn in the same interdose interval, a possibly different interval for each individual. The number of this interval, n_j, was chosen randomly with equal probability from the set (1, 2, 3, 5). The set of sampling times in this interval is chosen randomly with equal probability from the set of (0.2, 0.4, 0.6, 1.0) of size m_j. A sample at time 1.0 was assumed to be taken immediately prior to the next dose. For the baseline data set, the basic design is used with $m_j = 2$ for all j, n = 50.

Because "true" parameter values are known in the simulations, the degree of bias and the precision of the parameter estimates provided by each method can be compared. For each simulation, 30 replications of complete data sets were analyzed and for each kth replication (of the 30), the percentage error, %E(k), for each estimate was calculated. In the case of clearance, the %E(k) was

$$\%E(k) = \frac{Cl(k) - Cl}{Cl} \bullet 100 \qquad \text{(Eq. 2)}$$

where Cl = (true) population value (0.693 herein) and Cl(k) = estimate of clearance at the kth replication by some method. An estimate of the bias of the method's estimator of clearance is the average %E(k) denoted %E. The statistical significance of the difference of %E from zero was tested with the *t*-test. An estimate of the precision of the method's estimator of clearance is the standard deviation of the %E(k), denoted %SDE.

Results. Figures 2–5 illustrate the results from the various simulations. Bias and precision of the population parameter estimates are indicated by the shaded bars for the STS method and by the open bars for the NONMEM method. The ordinate is in units of percentage error (%E) as defined by Equation 2. The average %E is indicated by the horizontal line in the middle of the bar corresponding to the parameter and the method. Significant (p < 0.05) biases are indicated by asterisks in the bars. The full height of each bar is two standard deviations of the %E. This measures the precision of the estimator. Each panel shows the results for each population parameter for both methods. The parameters for Cl, clearance; V_d, volume of distribution; σ_{Cl}, interindividual coefficient of variation of Cl; σ_{V_d}, interindividual coefficient of variation of V_d; and σ_e, the coefficient of variation of residual error.

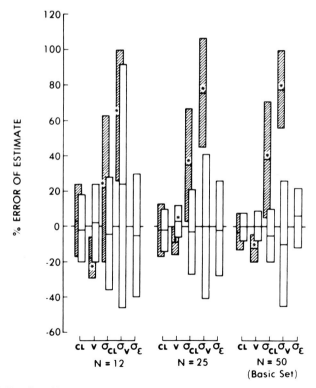

Figure 2. The effect of increasing population size. See text for format. The three panels show results for data like that of the basic design, but using 12, 25, and (the basic set itself) 50 individuals (reprinted with permission from Reference 12).

Effect of Increasing n. The usefulness of NONMEM is based on the premise that a limited number of samples from a large population of patients can be used to accurately and precisely estimate population pharmacokinetic parameters. The question then becomes, ''What is the optimal number of subjects to include in such a study?''

Figure 2 shows the results of the analysis of the basic data set (n = 50) and the effect of reducing the population to 25 and 12 individuals. As noted by Sheiner and Beal, as n increases, the precision of the estimates of both methods also increases. However, the biases for the STS method do not tend to decrease, confirming the inconsistency of the estimates of the method for V_d and for the interindividual random-effect parameters. They further state that the analysis of the basic data set (n = 50) using the STS method results in a significant downwards bias in the estimate of V_d, and very large upwards bias in the estimate of the interindividual random-effect parameters.[12] None of the NONMEM estimates show significant bias, although the poor precision of the estimate of σ_{V_d} inhibits the detection of even moderate bias. The upward bias in the STS estimates of σ_{Cl} and σ_{V_d} is due to first-stage estimation error, as discussed previously.

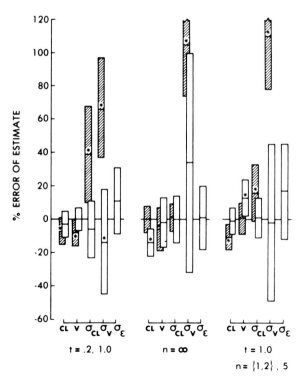

Figure 3. The effect of sampling design. See text for format. The three panels show results for different data designs. In the first, only peak and trough samples are taken. In the second, all samples are taken at steady state. In the last, only trough samples are taken, one from the fifth dose interval and one from the first or second interval (reprinted with permission from Reference 12).

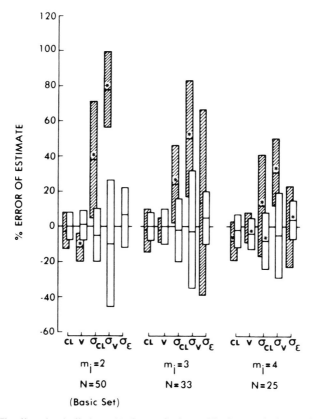

Figure 4. The effect of tradeoff of n vs. M_j. See text for format. The three panels show results for data like that from the basic design and with the same number of data points per data set (100). In the first panel, there are 2 points from each of 50 individuals (the basic set); in the second, 3 points from each of 33 individuals; and in the third, 4 points from each of 25 individuals (reprinted with permission from Reference 12).

If, as suggested by Sheiner and Beal, a parameter estimate is acceptably precise with %SDE ≤ 20 percent, then under the basic design, such precision is achieved at n = 25 for both fixed effect parameters.[12] However, even at n = 50, the %SDE of the estimate of σ_{V_d} (by NONMEM) considerably exceeds 20 percent and that of σ_{Cl} is still 15 percent. The problem of precisely estimating components of variance has been discussed previously.[4] The results of this simulation suggest that the minimum number of patients to be included in a population pharmacokinetic study is 50, particularly if an estimate of interindividual variability is of interest.

Effect of Sampling Design. True routine clinical data are generally characterized by a lack of design in the sampling scheme. It is possible, however, to exert some control over the pattern of sampling. Figure 3 shows the results of three such sampling protocols. In each case, two samples were obtained from each individual and 50 subjects were included.[12]

In the first panel, only peak and trough levels were obtained ($t = 0.2$ and $t = 1.0$). The second panel shows the results of only sampling at steady state, and the third panel shows the results of a sampling design in which only trough levels are obtained. For this last design, one trough level was obtained at steady state, and the other trough level was obtained following either the first or second dose.[12]

As discussed by Sheiner and Beal, the peak and trough results (first panel, Figure 3) are very similar to the basic set results for either method (third panel, Figure 2). Their conclusion is that a more careful design of sampling times to increase the difference between concentrations in an interdose interval yields relatively little benefit.[12]

The results for steady-state sampling (second panel, Figure 3) show some differences from the basic set results particularly in regard to V_d. The STS estimates of Cl and σ_{Cl} are more precise, while both STS and NONMEM estimates of V_d and σ_{V_d} are less precise. As pointed out by Sheiner and Beal, this reflects the relative lack of information regarding V_{dj} in steady-state data and the corresponding greater information regarding Cl_j.[12]

The results of the trough-only sampling design (third panel, Figure 3) as compared to the basic set results show greater precision for both

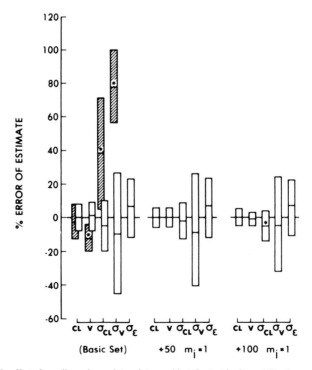

Figure 5. The effect of sampling only one data point per subject. See text for format. The three panels show results when one-point-per-individual data are used. In the first panel the results for the basic data set, using only two-points-per-individual data, are shown. In the second panel NONMEM results are shown for the basic data set plus an additional 50 one-point-per-individual points. In the third panel, 100 one-point-per-individual points are added to the basic data set (reprinted with permission from Reference 12).

the STS and NONMEM estimates of Cl and σ_{Cl} and poorer precision for estimates of V_d and σ_{V_d} by both methods. According to Sheiner and Beal, this illustrates the problem of estimating V_d from the rate of attainment of steady state, rather than from the rate of decay of Cp with time.[12]

The results of these three simulation studies suggest that one should exert minimal control over the sampling scheme employed in collecting population pharmacokinetic data. One should attempt, however, to obtain data under a variety of circumstances; i.e., steady state and nonsteady state, peak, trough, and midpoint levels should all be included.

Number of Subjects vs. Number of Samples per Subject. Figure 4 shows the results of the effect of varying the number of individuals (n) and the number of drug levels obtained per subject (m). In the basic data set, 2 levels were obtained from 50 individuals. The second simulation allows 3 drug levels from each of 33 individuals, and the third simulation allows 4 from each of 25 individuals.[12]

The results of these simulations suggest that for the STS method, the tradeoff favors more samples per individual. The bias in its estimate of V_d decreases, and the upward bias in the interindividual random effect parameters decreases. As noted by the authors, the latter is expected, as estimation error in V_{dj} and Cl_j decreases as m_j increases. Note also that the STS estimate of $\sigma\epsilon$ (now available) is not very precise. Their conclusion regarding NONMEM is very different. No loss is incurred with NONMEM using fewer data points per individual. As few as two data points per subject can be used to estimate the major population pharmacokinetic parameters of interest. This provides further evidence that NONMEM is capable of taking advantage of routine clinical data.[12]

One Sample per Subject. The final simulation takes this a step further and investigates the value of using the ultimate in sparse data, a single data point from an individual. As described by Sheiner and Beal, the basic data set was augmented with data from 50 individuals, each with $m_j = 1$ (the data were generated using the same procedure for randomly selecting n_{ij} and t_{ij} as with the basic set). This augmented data set was then analyzed by NONMEM for the population parameters. Next, the augmented data set was further augmented with data from another 50 individuals, each with $m_j = 1$, and the entire set was reanalyzed.[12]

The results shown in Figure 5 indicate that NONMEM can take advantage of $m_j = 1$ data to improve the precision of its estimates of all the population parameters with the possible exception of $\sigma\epsilon$.[12]

Analysis of Clinical Trial Data—Alprazolam

Although simulations are useful in examining the behavior of a data analysis approach, knowledge of the performance of a method when analyzing data from a clinical trial is also needed. In order to gain some insight into this question, a population pharmacokinetic analysis using data obtained during a multiple dosing trial of alprazolam was performed. The objectives of this study were to (1) empirically compare NONMEM to the STS method, and (2) evaluate the ability to utilize fragmentary amounts of data per individual using NONMEM. This was accomplished by repeating the analysis of the data using progressively smaller amounts of data per subject. The material in this section summarizes this study.[13]

METHODS

Ten healthy, adult male subjects, mean weight (SD) 79.9 (44.4) kg, were initially given alprazolam 1 mg po, followed by 0.5 mg po q8h for seven days. Seventeen alprazolam plasma concentrations were obtained during the 48 hours after the first and last doses. In addition, 12 trough levels were obtained from each subject during the multiple dosing period (Figure 6).

Population pharmacokinetic parameters of alprazolam were obtained using the following methods.

STS Method. For this approach, the alprazolam concentrations obtained after the first and last dose were used. In the first stage, clearance was estimated after the first and last dose by dividing the dose by the appropriate area under the plasma concentration-time curve (AUC). The elimination rate constant (k_e) was estimated by least-squares regression analysis of the terminal log-linear decay phase. The apparent volume of distribution (V_d) was then calculated as the ratio of clearance and the elimination rate constant. The estimates of clearance, k_e, and V_d for each individual were the means of the values obtained after the first and last dose.

In the second stage, the population parameters were estimated by taking the mean of the corresponding individual estimates. In light of the pharmacostatistical model used for the NONMEM analysis, the geometric mean of the individual estimates was used. Estimates of the

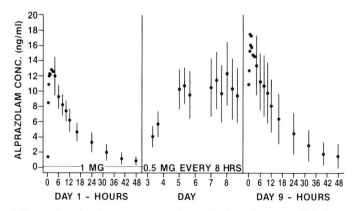

Figure 6. Average alprazolam plasma concentration-time profile observed with the multiple-dose regimen; (+) represents mean (± 1 SD) alprazolam concentrations. Alprazolam concentrations measured after first and last dose used for STS approach. Trough levels drawn on days 3 through 8 used for NONMEM analysis (reprinted with permission from Reference 13).

Table 1. Comparison of Methods for Estimating
Population Pharmacokinetic Parameters of Alprazolam

	TWO-STAGE	NONMEM		
		DATA-1	DATA-2	DATA-3
Number of subjects	10	10	10	10
Number of samples per subject	36	12	6	3
Clearance (L/h/kg) (CI)	0.060* (0.03–0.12)	0.060 (0.047–0.073)	0.059 (0.050–0.068)	0.060 (0.049–0.070)
Coefficient of Variation (CI)	0.29 (NA)	0.29 (0.16–0.39)	0.27 (0.17–0.34)	0.28 (0.17–0.36)
V_d (L/kg) (CI)	1.05* (0.84–1.32)	1.56 (1.2–1.9)	1.37 (1.1–1.6)	1.53 (1.1–1.9)
Coefficient of Variation (CI)	0.14 (NA)	0.45 (0.16–0.62)	0.47 (0–0.82)	0.84 (0–1.45)
k_e (h^{-1}) (CI)	0.058* (0.031–0.108)	0.038† (0.028–0.048)	0.044† (0.035–0.053)	0.039† (0.031–0.046)
Coefficient of Variation (CI)	0.28 (NA)	0.54 (NC)	0.55 (NC)	0.89 (NC)

CI = 95 percent confidence interval; NA = not available; NC = not calculated.
*Geometric mean.
†Calculated from estimates of Cl and V_d.

interindividual random-effect parameters were obtained by calculating the standard deviations of the logs of the corresponding fixed-effect parameters. A confidence interval for each fixed effect parameter is obtained from the exponentials of the endpoints of the usual 95 percent confidence interval for a mean computed from the logs of the individual estimates. There is no appropriate method to compute 95 percent confidence intervals for random interindividual effect parameters.[4,13]

NONMEM. The 12 trough levels obtained from each subject during the multiple-dosing trial were combined and analyzed with NONMEM using a one-compartment model with first-order elimination. Drug absorption was modeled as a zero-order infusion process over a 1.5-hour period, the average time to peak obtained in previous studies.[14] The bioavailability in both cases was assumed to be unity (data on file, Upjohn Company, Kalamazoo, MI). This simple pharmacokinetic model was required because of the nature of the sampling scheme: only trough levels were available. In order to further evaluate the ability to estimate population pharmacokinetic parameters from fragmentary data, the number of trough levels for each subject was progressively reduced by randomly removing trough levels from each individual. In this fashion, three data sets were created. The original data set contained 12 trough levels per subject (data-1), a second data set contained 6 trough levels per subject (data-2), and a third data set contained 3 trough levels per subject (data-3). Ten subjects were included in each data set. Estimates of population pharmacokinetic parameters of alprazolam were obtained for each data set using NONMEM.[13]

RESULTS

Table 1 summarizes the results obtained in this study. The estimate of the population mean clearance obtained using the STS approach, 0.06 L/h/kg, is identical to the estimate of clearance obtained using NONMEM. The 95 percent confidence interval for the NONMEM approach is narrower, however. Note that the NONMEM parameter estimates remain stable even as the number of samples is reduced from 12 to 6 to 3 per subject. The estimates of the coefficient of variation for clearance are also similar for the two methods.

The estimate of the population mean V_d obtained using the STS approach is 1.1 L/kg, whereas the corresponding NONMEM estimates are somewhat higher (1.56 L/kg, 1.37, and 1.53 for data-1, data-2, and data-3, respectively). With the exception of data-3, the NONMEM-calculated 95 percent confidence intervals were narrower than calculated with the STS approach. Moreover, the estimates of the coefficient of variation of V_d obtained using NONMEM are also higher (45, 47, and 84 percent for data-1, data-2, and data-3, respectively) than the corresponding estimate of 14 percent obtained using the STS approach. Also, note that the NONMEM-calculated 95 percent confidence interval for this parameter is rather large and increases as the amount of data decreases.[13]

The estimate of the elimination rate constant, k_e, obtained using the STS approach parameter estimates of Cl and V_d, is 0.055 h^{-1}. The values for k_e, obtained using NONMEM's estimates of Cl and V_d, are 0.038, 0.044, and 0.039 for data-1, data-2, and data-3, respectively.

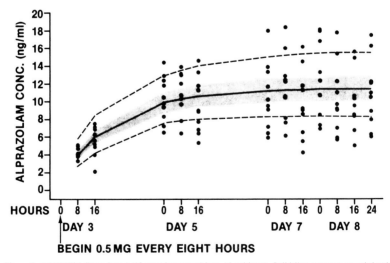

Figure 7. NONMEM fit to data-1 (12 samples per subject, 10 subjects). Solid line connects trough levels predicted for mean individual in the study (79.9 kg male) using population pharmacokinetic parameters obtained with NONMEM. The shaded area represents ± 1 SD of intraindividual variability. The area bounded by the dashed lines represents ± 1 SD of both inter- and intraindividual variability (reprinted with permission from Reference 13).

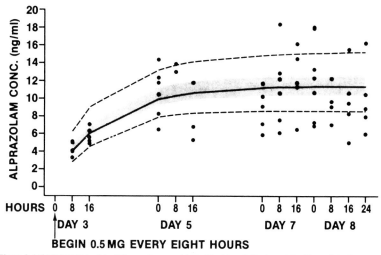

Figure 8. NONMEM fit to data-2 (6 samples per subject, 10 subjects). See legend for Figure 7 for interpretation (reprinted with permission from Reference 13).

Figures 7–9 illustrate the fit to the data using the population pharmacokinetic parameters obtained with NONMEM.[13]

DISCUSSION

The results obtained for V_d in this study are expected given the results of the simulation discussed above (see Figure 3, panel 3). The higher estimates for V_d and the larger 95 percent confidence intervals are undoubtedly the result of the sampling scheme. Most of the samples were obtained at steady state and very few samples were obtained during the accumulation of steady state. Thus, very little information is available regarding V_d.

It is difficult to assess the estimates of interindividual variability obtained by either method in this study. Although the NONMEM-generated parameter estimates have been shown to be relatively unbiased, they are highly imprecise (see Figure 3, panels 2 and 3).[12]

Guidelines for Study Design

Based on the results of the simulation studies and the alprazolam population study discussed above, we can begin to develop guidelines that can be used in setting up population pharmacokinetic studies for NONMEM analysis.

1. Samples should be obtained at random time points from each individual and not according to a rigid experimental protocol. As demonstrated by the above studies, the commonly employed method of obtaining only trough levels during multiple-dosing trials is unnecessarily restrictive and limits the information that can be extracted from the data.

2. A minimum of two to four samples should be obtained from each subject, depending on the number of pharmacokinetic parameters to be estimated. As described previously, however, data consisting of only one sample per subject are capable of supplying additional information when combined with more extensive data.

3. A minimum of 50 subjects should be included, and the population should comprise patients who are representative of the population who take the drug therapeutically. This will ensure that a representative sample of patients is included and improve the estimates of interindividual variability.

4. Subjects can be receiving a variety of concomitant medications and diet should not be restricted. Careful analysis of this data can provide information on a variety of possible drug-drug and drug-food interactions.

5. Complete demographic data, i.e., age, weight, height, sex, and concomitant disease states, should be collected on all patients. This will allow investigations into the effect of these factors on drug disposition.

Summary

Under the current system of drug development and approval, traditional pharmacokinetic studies are performed and results are used to obtain population pharmacokinetic parameters. These parameters are then used to develop the initial dosing guidelines included in the package insert. Depending on the availability of therapeutic drug monitoring, subsequent adjustment of drug dosage may be made based on

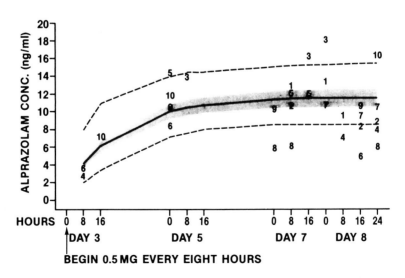

Figure 9. NONMEM fit to data-3 (3 samples per subject, 10 subjects). See legend for Figure 7 for interpretation. Numbers identify samples belonging to specific individuals (reprinted with permission from Reference 13).

measured drug concentrations in the patient. Unfortunately, in most cases, the feedback obtained from this process is not further exploited.

Guidelines for population-specific dosing adjustments are not generally available until a clinically significant disaster occurs and the patient population involved is intensively studied. Thus, inappropriate dosing recommendations may not be detected for a significant period of time, if at all.

NONMEM represents a tool that can be used to analyze the data generated during the routine clinical care of patients and, if employed systematically, could allow problems to be detected at an early stage of drug development before irreversible damage to patients or the reputation of the drug has occurred.

References

1. SHEINER LB, ROSENBERG B, MARATHE VV. Estimation of population characteristics of pharmacokinetic parameters from routine clinical data. *J Pharmacokinet Biopharm* 1977;5:445-79.

2. SHEINER LB, BEAL SL. Bayesian individualization of pharmacokinetics: simple implementation and comparison with non-Bayesian methods. *J Pharm Sci* 1982;71:1344-8.

3. SHEINER LB, BEAL SL. Evaluation of methods for estimating population pharmacokinetic parameters. I. Michaelis-Menten model: routine clinical pharmacokinetic data. *J Pharmacokinet Biopharm* 1980;8:553-71.

4. SHEINER LB, BEAL SL. Evaluation of methods for estimating population pharmacokinetic parameters. II. Biexponential model and experimental pharmacokinetic data. *J Pharmacokinet Biopharm* 1981;9:635-51.

5. SHEINER LB, BEAL SL. Estimation of pooled pharmacokinetic parameters describing populations. In: Endrenyi L, ed. Kinetic data analysis, design and analysis of enzyme and pharmacokinetic experiments. New York: Plenum Press, 1981:271-83.

6. SHEINER LB. Drug dosage: forecasting and control for a target level strategy. In: Wilkinson GR, Rowland M, eds. Drug disposition and metabolism. Lancaster, England: MTP Press Limited, 1985:211-50.

7. JENNRICH RT, SAMPSON PF. Newton-Raphson and related algorithms for maximum likelihood variance component estimation. *Technometrics* 1976;18:11-7.

8. GRASELA TH, SHEINER LB. Population pharmacokinetics of procainamide from routine clinical data. *Clin Pharmacokinet* 1984;9:545-54.

9. GRASELA TH, SHEINER LB, RAMBECK B, et al. Steady-state pharmacokinetics of phenytoin from routinely collected patient data. *Clin Pharmacokinet* 1983;8:355-64.

10. GRASELA TH, DONN SM. Neonatal population pharmacokinetics of phenobarbital derived from routine clinical data. *Dev Pharmacol Ther* 1985;8:374-83.

11. MUNGALL DR, LUDDEN TM, MARSHALL J, et al. Population pharmacokinetics of warfarin. *J Pharmacokinet Biopharm* 1985;13:213-27.

12. SHEINER LB, BEAL SL. Evaluation of methods for estimating population pharmacokinetic parameters. III. Monoexponential model: routine clinical data. *J Pharmacokinet Biopharm* 1983;11:303-19.

13. GRASELA TH, ANTAL EJ, TOWNSEND RJ, SMITH RB. An evaluation of population pharmacokinetics in therapeutic trials. Part 1. Comparison of methodologies. *Clin Pharmacol Ther* 1986;39:605-12.

14. BEAL SL, SHEINER LB. The NONMEM system. *Am Statistician* 1980:34:118-9.

8. SYMPOSIUM SUMMARY

Randy P. Juhl

IN THIS SYMPOSIUM we have viewed the continuing evolution of pharmacokinetic and pharmacodynamic studies from several perspectives. I would like to thank the speakers for sharing with us their mistakes as well as their considerable discoveries. It is exciting and interesting to view the increased interaction between those with clinical and kinetic backgrounds and the continued evolution of our abilities to pursue knowledge through our research.

As stated in the introduction to this symposium, the types of investigations that were discussed are not new. Many of the problems and challenges are of long standing. What is new however, is the increasing number of scientists who are performing such studies. Investigator demographics are also changing as the research interests of clinical pharmacists and pharmacokineticists continue to overlap. I believe that this interaction gives those of us in pharmacy a greatly enhanced potential for continued impact on drug research issues.

Along with an increased potential to contribute, we also should feel the real burden of responsibility to direct our efforts in a cost-effective manner. Because both our financial and human resources are finite and at times even scarce, we must carefully select areas of investigation and rigorously define the methods of inquiry. The latter is accomplished through careful attention to study design. Recognizing and controlling potential sources of variability is the cardinal element of study design; and study design is the single most important component of research activity. The emergence of pharmacodynamic investigation presents a whole new set of variables that must be considered. The speakers have defined the preferred approach for several important research functions and have also pointed out errors and shortcomings made by other investigators as well as some they made themselves. In doing so, they have admirably achieved the goal of this symposium.